FLIPSIDE

FLIPSIDE

A TOURIST'S GUIDE
ON HOW TO NAVIGATE
THE AFTERLIFE

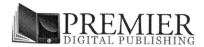

Premier Digital Publishing, Los Angeles

PREFACE

"You can't always get what you want, but if you try sometimes, you just might find, you get what you need."

- Mick Jagger & Keith Richards

An ad came on television of a beautiful young model wearing a skimpy bra and angel wings. She was dancing provocatively, selling the latest in underwear for Victoria's Secret. My 3 year old son stood up and pointed excitedly at the television. "Daddy!" he said, staring at the model and then looking at me. "I want that!"

I chuckled, remembering that he'd once told me that he remembered being a monk in a past life. "But RJ," I protested, "I thought you were a monk." "Not anymore!" he said happily.

CONTENTS

FOREWORD

"Is life designed in advance? Are we all part of some elaborately plotted mini-series that runs every waking moment? Does it really matter one way or the other? We're on the planet for a reason, we have roles to play, we might as well play them as well as we can. However, that doesn't prevent me from perennially rooting for the Cubs."

Richard Martini, author of *FlipSide*.

Is there a greater spiritual reality? Does consciousness survive physical death? Are past lives real? Is there a creative grand plan – some sort of a Divine Plot – of which we are all a part, and can we individually and collectively contribute to *It's* design and unfolding? And assuming for the moment some sort of a grand planning process exists, the question arises; does *It* – whom I have come to think of as being an "Infinite Teacher" – have a sense of humor?

I am scientist by training and profession. My laboratory research has led me to address these kinds of questions in various books including *The Afterlife Experiments, The G.O.D. Experiments,* and *The Sacred Promise.* Like Richard Martini, the author of *FlipSide,* I am a skeptic in the core sense of this word – meaning a wonderer, a questioner, and a genuine seeker of truth.

Of all these great questions, the hypothesis of past lives – the continued re-living of individual souls for the sake of our learning and evolving – is among the least researched and most controversial. The truth is, science knows virtually nothing about the concept of incarnation or consciousness. Contemporary science simply assumes the idea of incarnation is a myth (and a fallacious one at that), and according to mainstream neuroscience, consciousness is an emergent property of neural networks, an evolutionary side effect so to speak of the invention of the brain and nervous system.

According to the prevailing views of mainstream science, there can be no such thing as the incarnation of consciousness because the brain is the sole creator of consciousness. Most neuroscientists don't entertain the hypothesis the brain might be a brilliantly designed antenna and receiver for consciousness which somehow returns – incarnates and/or connects (for example, resonates) with the brain.

An emerging body of consciousness research (typically classified under the umbrella of parapsychology), when combined with contemporary quantum physics, seriously challenges the belief the brain is the creator of consciousness. This new evidence requires we reconsider the idea of the incarnation of consciousness, and by extension, the plausibility (if not probability) of reincarnation. Three types of scientific inquiry together can provide us with important evidence which addresses these great questions:

Type I Self-Science: Evidence obtained in the laboratories of our individual lives, where personal observations are recorded and examined from a skeptical (questioning), science-oriented frame of mind.

Type II Exploratory Investigations: Where scientists use themselves as preliminary prototype subjects, testing new laboratory methods and procedures on themselves, and

Type III Conventional Research: When controlled experiments are conducted on human or animal subjects following federal and university rules and guidelines.

Although Type III Conventional Research is the most respected and sometimes the most definitive, Type I Self-Science is often where the most innovative and core discoveries are made. The history of science reminds us that great scientists like Isaac Newton and Albert Einstein took Type I observations made in their personal lives and successfully translated them into revolutionary Type III theories and discoveries. When these three types of evidence collectively come to the same conclusion, their combined impact is significantly greater than either one alone.

Richard Martini's *FlipSide* is an inspiring and well written – as well as entertaining – journey of Type I Self-Science which is focused on the interrelated questions of (1) reincarnation and past lives, (2) past life regression and healing, and (3) the existence of a universal grand designer and plan.

As you read Richard's journey of personal discovery in the context of these great questions, you will awaken to a vision of mind and the universe which is filled with opportunity and awe. This is the kind of the book where once you have read it, you will no longer be able to see the world in the same way again.

I must confess that after reading *FlipSide,* it appears that I may no longer be able to resist bringing past life hypothesis research into the laboratory. Though this book has not resulted in my deciding to root for the Cubs (smile), it has encouraged me to root for the possibility that Richard's observations and insights will prove to be valid and meaningful for all of us.

Gary E. Schwartz, PhD[1]

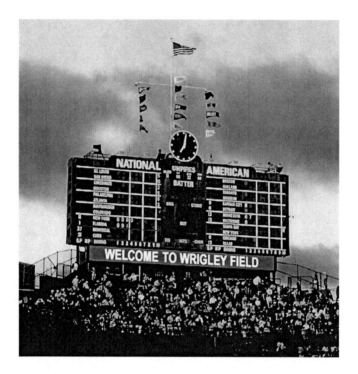

"We have no reliable guarantee that the afterlife will be any less exasperating than this one, have we?"

- Noel Coward

[1]   Gary E. Schwartz, PhD is a professor of psychology, medicine, neurology, psychiatry, and surgery, and Director of the Laboratory for Advances in Health at the University of Arizona. He received his PhD from Harvard University, was a professor of psychiatry and psychology at Yale University as well as Director of the Yale Psychophysiology Center and co-director of the Yale Behavioral Medicine Clinic from 1976-1988. His books include *The Afterlife Experiments, The G.O.D. Experiments, The Energy Healing Experiments,* and *The Sacred Promise.*

INTRODUCTION

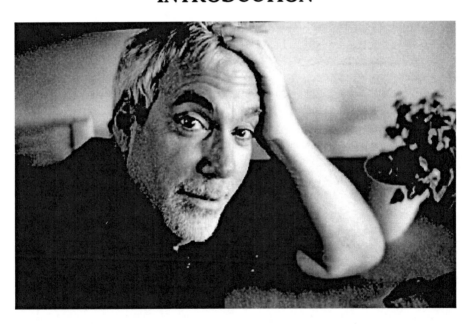

Skeptic. n. 1. One who instinctively or habitually doubts, questions, or disagrees with assertions or generally accepted conclusions. One who is yet undecided as to what is true; one who is looking or inquiring for what is true; an inquirer after facts or reasons.[2]

I consider myself a skeptic in the truest sense of the word. I've always been wary of the accepted norms of how the world works, at least how everyone else has agreed over millennia what those norms are. My friend and mentor, film director

---

[2] American Heritage Dictionary and www.dictionary.net/sceptic

Phillip Noyce, not without a touch of irony, recently said of me with his Sydney accent "Richard has a penchant for looking into mysteries that defy resolution." [3]

A bit of my background: Irish-Italian, third generation immigrant. I was raised Catholic, attend a Presbyterian church, journeyed into the heart of Buddhism through India and Tibet, and consider myself a spiritualist – appreciative of all religious backgrounds and insight. I'm a free-lance journalist, have written or directed a number of feature films and documentaries, and have worked for some of the great writer-directors of cinema including Noyce and Robert Towne.

I mention this in passing because inevitably it's pointed out I have no expertise in *any* particular field -- other than being open to following an interesting story. If you're interested in just what experts have to say on this controversial subject, I humbly recommend reading someone else. That being said, I was thrilled when Gary E. Schwartz, who received his PhD from Harvard University, was a professor of psychiatry and psychology at Yale University as well as Director of the Yale Psychophysiology Center and co-director of the Yale Behavioral Medicine Clinic offered to write the Foreword to *FlipSide*. "Self science," he writes, "is where core discoveries are made." I may not be a scientist, but I know someone who is.

It was the death and subsequent visitation from my closest friend that prompted my journey into the afterlife. She appeared one afternoon, after her death, to guide me to the location where she now resides. How could that be? Either I imagined it, or she actually had taken me to her location in "another galaxy." The event started the journey into the afterlife, if only to see if I could find her again, on my own.

I began with a documentary about reincarnation, planning to cover both sides of the issue - the science of doubt and the religion of belief. I investigated past life regression through the work of Dr. Brian Weiss, Ian Stevenson of the University of Virginia, and Carol Bowman. Along the path, I learned of the work of Dr. Michael Newton, a hypnotherapist who'd done over 7000 sessions with clients under "deep hypnosis;" these sessions revealed not only previous lives, but a place *between lives* where everyone learns how and why we return for another lifetime on Earth.

This book looks beyond past life regression, reincarnation, religion, psychics or ESP, giving new perspective on these disciplines in light of the groundbreaking Life Between Life research. It demonstrates that most past life regressions don't go deep enough, the study of reincarnation doesn't go far enough, Psychics are unable give their clients an opportunity to really see their unfiltered selves, and most religions dismiss what people say about experiences with the spirit world if they're contrary to their tenets. And the scientific community's strict adherence to a belief that all memories of past lives or life between lives is Cryptomnesia, or entirely made up is, at the very least, near-sighted. After all, no one in the world of science has yet been able to clearly define consciousness.

---

[3] Phillip Noyce, director of "Salt" "Rabbit Proof Fence" and "Clear and Present Danger."

According to Dr. Newton's extensive research, this "Life between Lives" realm is inaccessible to our conscious mind, but through deep hypnosis (and as we'll see in this book, through other experiences, near death or consciousness altering incidents) we can return there to learn why we *chose our parents, chose our life's path*, or our very *reason for existence on the planet.*

Newton's work presents an either-or dichotomy; two people who don't know each other claiming to say the same things under hypnosis about the afterlife would be worth examining. But thousands? Either Newton had influenced patients through leading questions, (false memories, or remembrance of overhearing someone else's tale) or what they were saying was true.

"People cannot really be lead into histories of their past lives or life between lives," Dr. Newton wrote in a follow up email. "Even if a subject were somehow able to overcome hypnosis and construct a fantasy about the spirit world--or free associate with prior conceptions--their biased responses would be inconsistent with all of my other cases. I had thousands of cases before I wrote a single word for my first book. It did not matter if my clients were atheists or religious fundamentalists; once I had them in deep hypnosis they all told me basically the same things concerning the spirit world and their life after death."

The same things about life after death. Thousands who never met reporting the same thing about the Afterlife; how could that possibly be?

The only verbal direction I've heard Newton or his protégés give a client is to *"Be there now."* That basic directive encourages people to see beyond conscious life, into lives stored somewhere in our unconscious memories, (or reportedly stored in energy fields outside our physical bodies) and into a world that exists independent of time and space. His clients claimed they could access deceased loved ones; learn why they chose previous lives, why these chose *this* life, and how the two intersect. If I was going to find my deceased friend, then this was the place to begin.

I attended a conference where over 100 hypnotherapists from around the world had come to earn accreditation with The Newton Institute (TNI). To ensure a certain quality of candidates "All applicants must be accredited graduates of recognized hypnosis schools and have from 2 to 3 years practical experience in public practice,"[4] as well as submit an audio tape of a past life regression done with a client. While some of the students seemed more connected with a new age, crystal using, angels-over-your-shoulder genre, I met and interviewed many who felt *compelled* to the field, who had changed their life's path for reasons unbeknownst to them; as if called to the work by a higher power.

---

[4] As per an email from Dr. Newton about the requirements involved.

During the weeklong conference, candidates practice on each other doing past life regressions (PLRs) and life between life sessions. (LBLs) The volunteer session I attended was with a woman I'll call "Noreen," who is a working hypnotherapist in the Southwest. President of TNI, Paul Aurand, conducted the session, and Michael Newton sat nearby using a marker and large white board for making silent observations as the three hour session progressed.

By the time her session ended I felt the axis of the Earth shift. She had the same bullet points in her session that all of Newton's patients had, confirming what I'd read in the research. Still, was it possible the elaborate emotional exploration had been staged for my benefit and those in her class?

I attended and filmed a number of other sessions, all of them equally revelatory, and was able to interview the retired Dr. Newton for the last he'll give on the subject. I also interviewed his wife. "What did you think when your husband came home with these afterlife stories?" I asked. "I thought the men in white coats were going to cart him away," she said, candidly. However once she heard tapes of his sessions, she realized everyone was having the *same* experiences; "Complete strangers were saying identical things about the afterlife."

The Newton Institute offered me a session of my own. I'd never been under hypnosis before, am self-conscious as it is, especially when there's a camera involved, but in a George Plimpton-like moment, I realized I had to participate. I came away from my session feeling as if the Earth had further shifted on its axis. Everything I thought I knew was no longer operative. *I'd taken the red pill* as they say.

I can appreciate that being LA-based, or being a spiritual seeker myself makes my "willingness to believe" suspect, or less than surprising. But my career has trained me to disbelieve, and it's the copious amount of evidence presented within that has convinced me otherwise. I can't help that I chose Richard Martini as my vehicle for this life, but in light of this research, I see that the complex and clever journey to find it is pretty much the way it was evidently planned in advance. But I'm a skeptic in the true sense of the word: *One who is yet undecided as to what is true.*

In this book, I'm going to demonstrate how we all can make this same journey to a life between lives, and discover the very reasons for our existence on earth. Answering these questions is the central and exciting premise of this book; there is dramatic and new evidence of life before and after death, and with proper guidance any one of us can travel there and learn why we chose previous lives, and *how and why* we chose our current one.

So please, sit back and relax, allow me to guide you on this unusual trip into another realm.

But buckle up; it's going to be a bumpy ride.

"If there is reincarnation, I'd like to come back as Warren Beatty's fingertips."

- Woody Allen

CHAPTER 1
LUANA'S ASHES

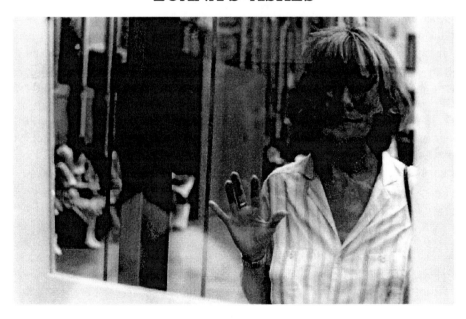

"I have this recurring dream where I'm in another dimension in a room full of spiritual beings, all dressed in white, and a teacher is speaking to me in a language I've never heard before, but I absolutely understand everything he is saying... - I think I'm on my way to another galaxy."

- Luana Anders, actress/writer, just prior to her passing in July 1996.

Fade in: Day. A bedroom bathed in light. Two old friends talking, one friend paralyzed, in bed. The other friend hears her speaking and looks down from his newspaper. "You're going where?" My best friend and 20 year companion, Luana,[1] was lying paralyzed in her bed in her home town, Mar Vista, California, telling me that she had this recurring dream that she was going to a classroom in another galaxy.

Luana had been diagnosed with terminal breast cancer. I had the unfortunate task of watching my pal dissipate in body over the last two years of her life. When I wanted to take her for an adventure, I'd pick her up and carry her to the car, and we'd take a trip for cappuccino somewhere - a treat she never tired of enjoying. I felt it my honor and privilege to spend those last months and days with her - truthfully, I wouldn't be writing this book if I hadn't.

Luana had a profound influence on pretty much everyone she met. She acted in over 30 feature films, from "Easy Rider," to "Wild Bill," and over 300 televisions appearances, from "Dragnet," to "One Step Beyond." She was an actor's actor; she was close friends with Jack Nicholson, Robert Towne, Dennis Hopper, Sally Kellerman, Charles Grodin and others. She forged a lifelong friendship with a director who cast her in one of his first feature films "Dementia 13"; Francis Coppola. She made friends in all walks of life. Born in Mar Vista California, she'd been a bike messenger at MGM along with Nicholson, and they remained lifelong pals; Jack mentioned her passing when he accepted his Oscar for "As Good As It Gets."

Having become a Buddhist early in her career, she performed a Buddhist ceremony with Randy Quaid in "The Last Detail," written by her friend Robert Towne, starring her pal Jack Nicholson. I met her in a screenwriting class at USC film school. We were assigned a screenplay to examine together, and that led to a 20 year relationship. Despite an age difference between us - I was younger; it never seemed to be much of an issue between us. However, we did break up midway through our twenty years, and much to my relief, she opted to remain my close friend for the next ten years. One of her friends suggested her ensuing breast cancer might have been caused by our splitting up; she told him, "No, actually, Richard's the closest friend I have on the planet." I was honored to know her. Her influence on me was profound, and continues to reverberate as I write this sentence.

Watching a loved one pass may be the single most difficult thing we can do in life, and yet in some ways the most life enhancing, life changing event. I asked where she wanted me to scatter her ashes. She looked at me with her penetrating blue grey eyes and smiled. "Everywhere you go," she replied simply.

---

[1]   IMDB: Luana Anders or LuanaAnders.com

Just like her to give me a lifelong task. And I've lived it for the past 15 years, taking a little bit of her ashes wherever I go; I find an idyllic spot along a riverbank, across a bridge, I'll deposit a bit of her into the swirling waters below and say a hello to the planet on her behalf. Her ashes are in some amazing places, from the pond at the Guggenheim Museum designed by her pal Frank Gehry in Bilbao, to the small creek that runs behind the Dalai Lama's home in Dharamsala, from the fountains in front of the Vatican to the reflecting ponds in front of the Taj Mahal. From the waters in front of Sydney Opera house (where a rainbow appeared as I threw them) to the snowy trail around Mt. Kailash in Tibet to the great Chicago River, Luana is in a body of water somewhere near you.

She's in every state I've been, from Maine to Hawaii, in rivers like the Colorado, Chicago, Mississippi, Tiber, Arno, Seine, Thames, Brahmaputra, Sutlej, Ganges, Indus – in the Pacific, Atlantic, Indian Oceans, the Caribbean, Arabian, Mediterranean seas, in short, she's flowing in just about every water way I've visited in the past fifteen or so years since her passing. This girl gets around.

We never talked about death - everything was in a positive light, and we were battling together to try to dodge the inevitable bullet cancer can become. And despite any logic to the contrary, I agreed to help her as best I could through her journey. If she wanted to eschew traditional therapies, then I'd help her. If she wanted to get an MRI, we'd do that as well. It was arduous and her dearest friends stepped forward and helped her financially and emotionally through this Herculean task.

Then she told me she thought she was on her way to another galaxy.

It was a typical Sunday for us; I'd gone over with cappuccinos and a Sunday paper. She was too tired to read, and we talked and chuckled over the nonsense of the day, and she'd looked over a draft of a screenplay she was working on, something she did up until her last day on the planet. She poured herself into her work, and never let go of it. And then she casually mentioned she thought she was on her way "to another galaxy." I asked why.

She said, "I have this recurring dream; I'm in another galaxy, and we're in a classroom; everyone is dressed in white, it's a spiritual class of some kind, and the teacher is speaking to me in a language which I've never heard before, but completely understand." I nodded. Nothing I'd ever heard of before. A classroom? In another galaxy?

The day after she passed, I got a call from her lifelong friend Sandra,[2] who called from Hawaii. "I had this most amazing dream about her the other night. She was in a classroom, everyone was dressed in white, and she looked really happy." I thought that was a bit too coincidental, and I mentioned it to Luana's head nurse, Charmaine, a beautiful Caribbean woman who took care of her on a 24 hour basis. Charmaine nearly fainted. "That's the dream she kept having! She told me about it, she was in a classroom in another galaxy!"

---

[2] Sandra Stephenson, former actress who has become a spiritual life coach – infinitewaycoach.com

I mused Luana's class was probably hard to get into. Where I was in my life, my own spiritual journey, I thought that I'd never have enough credits to get in. But I also stored away the thought if I could figure out how to get into her class, I sure as hell would.

The night before Luana's passing, I had a number of unusual visions. I'd been spending days and nights with her, knowing from the hospice care nurses she wasn't long for this world. I was invited to a Hollywood party at a producer's home, and since Luana was resting comfortably, I thought I'd spend an hour or so unwinding, since the tension had been so great the past few weeks. I arrived at this soiree, and saw many of the Hollywood elite squiring beautiful people around on their arms. And then in flash, I saw them all in my friend's condition - frail, paralyzed, skin gaunt and pale, their last days on Earth. The vast crowd of people in designer clothes and red carpet dresses, in slow motion, all looking ancient and skeletal. It put a different perspective on the nature of fleeting beauty.

That night I slept at home, the first night I'd been away from her for a week. I was startled by a phone call at 3 in the morning. A gruff voice said "Yo, this is Tony. You paged me." I said "Sorry, wrong number," and hung up. I closed my eyes and put my head back on the pillow.

Suddenly the room was illuminated by the brightest light I've ever seen. My eyes were closed, but it was as if the roof of my building had disappeared and the light of a bright sun was shining down into my apartment. It was accompanied by the sound like an earthquake. It was a roar unlike anything I'd heard before, a combination of a massive freight train and the groaning of the Earth being formed.

I looked around and saw I was in some kind of volcano. The walls of the volcano were pulsating red, but I couldn't feel any heat. Above me was the shaft of light, and I was moving up towards it, scared out of my wits by what was happening. I had the conscious thought that I was on a platform moving up towards the opening, but then realized that I wasn't on it, but was actually part of it.

Then I heard Luana's voice, clear as a bell. "Isn't this fucking amazing?" The tone of her voice was younger, but distinctively hers. It was like her to throw "fuck" in a sentence when she was in her 20's, but quite unlike her to do so in her 50's. I then heard her say, "Isn't this unbelievable?"

I couldn't answer. The shaking, the light, the roar was so intense I lost consciousness. But when I came back moments later, I wasn't out of this vision; I was only higher along the journey. And as I neared the top, I had this odd feeling I could see between "channels" - the way old television sets looked between channels when you clicked them – halfway between the volcano, and some other place - another plane. Around me were sparks, like fireflies, crackling and sizzling with light. I had the wherewithal to say "I don't think I'm supposed to go here with you."

At that point, I lost consciousness again.

When I woke in the morning I was sure she had passed. I called the nurse at her home, and she said she hadn't, she was resting peacefully. I went over to her house to spend the day with her. As it turned out, it was her last one on Earth.

I called some of her friends to let them know she was passing. Lifelong friends Sally Kellerman and B.J. Merholz stopped by. Jack Nicholson, Robert Towne, Fred Roos and Charles Grodin called and said their goodbyes. The Coppolas called from Turkey to tell her how much they loved her and what a powerful force she'd been in their lives. She was lucky enough to say farewell to all those nearest and dearest to her.

Having been a Buddhist for 30 years, she belonged to a tight knit group of chanters who did "Gongyo" (she appeared in the film "The Last Detail" chanting for Randy Quaid) every day. I called a woman from her group, and she came to perform the parting ceremony for her. I could see Luana was pleased to have her friends show up like that, to pray for her. At some point they left, and I went in and held her hand. Her breath became shorter, and she turned to me and said, with determination; "Ha, ha, ha." She then passed away.

Or so I thought.

Her beloved cats were startled as they stared at the ceiling in unison, and then looked around the room as if following her spirit. The clocks in her home all stopped at 4 p.m.

Some weeks after her funeral ceremony, I took a job in New York City working for Charles Grodin on his CNBC show and was auditing Tibetan scholar Robert Thurman's class at Columbia University, when I got to see Luana again.

I was in my apartment on the upper west side one afternoon, overtired, and laid down to take a nap. I had been wondering where in the Universe Luana might be, if indeed she was still in our Universe.

As I drifted to sleep my body began vibrating and I could feel myself slipping out of it, like an out of body experience, which I'd had in the past a few times. But this was different. I shot out of my body like an arrow - I could see New York City disappearing below me, the way the Earth disappears in the film "Power of Ten," while traveling into outer space. I was traveling so fast the light of the stars blurred around me - not in the graphic way it happens in the Sci-Fi films, but similarly - and then suddenly I was tumbling and turning through what seemed like a worm hole, bouncing around at a high rate of speed until I was through the hole and into another galaxy - or another Universe perhaps. I was now traveling right to left instead of up and through, and suddenly I came to a halt, and I was standing a few inches from the face of Luana.

She opened her eyes and looked at me. There was no feeling of wonderment, or that I'd gone to heaven, or anything in particular - just a feeling of "You wanted to know where I was. Here I am."

And with that, a truck driver outside my window blasted his horn, as people are wont to do in the noisy New York afternoon, and oddly enough, I took the journey back, through the worm hole, back through space, back to the Earth zooming up to meet me and into my body - before the man's hand left the horn of his truck. Wow.

I felt as if I had found her in her "other galaxy" but where was it? When the film "Contact" came out, it included a journey into a worm hole, and as I watched it, I thought *that's it. That's the journey!* It wasn't like a dream; the experience was more visceral, as if I'd witnessed it. I'd gone to another galaxy without the benefit of a space suit.

Some years later, I was startled to open up Michael Newton's "Journey of Souls" and find people talking about classrooms in the afterlife. In yet another reference to them, I was in my local coffee shop when I asked a stranger why she named her daughter Krystal. "I've had this recurring dream that I'm in a classroom, and the teacher is dressed in white and works with energy. Then I'm in a room full of crystals."

Are these the same classrooms Luana and Michael Newton's clients were speaking of? As one friend of mine put it; "Oh no, we go to school for half of our lives as it is, I've got more classes to look forward to in the afterlife?"

But at least her classroom gave me a concrete place with which to begin this search for my dearly departed friend. The question became, how could I journey there to see her without 'kicking the bucket' myself? That became the focus of my quest, and ultimately the focus of this book; if our loved ones are out there, then where are they and how can we go to visit them? If there's life after death, and classrooms to boot, then where is the location of this campus? And by extension, if it's true we're eternal souls who reincarnate, what exactly is the process? And who's behind the master plan?

"To die will be an awfully big adventure."

- J.M. Barrie

CHAPTER 2
THE NEWTONIAN UNIVERSE

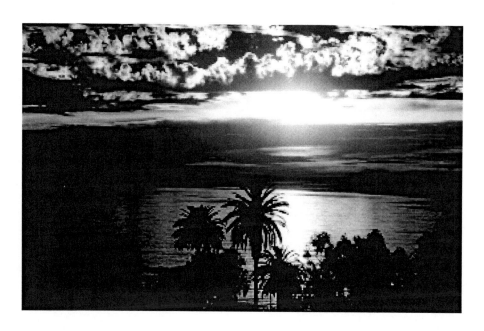

"I was like a boy playing on the sea-shore, and diverting myself now and then finding a smoother pebble or a prettier shell than ordinary, whilst the great ocean of truth lay all undiscovered before me."

- Sir Isaac Newton

As a therapeutic tool, hypnosis has been around for millennia. The ancient Greeks, Egyptians and Hindus all used forms of "Sleep Temples" to help people with various mental afflictions, and in 1207 Persian physician Avicenna (Ibn Sina) studied altered states where people could be both awake and asleep.[3] In 1841 British physician James Braid studied Eastern religious practices, including trances and deep meditation, and coined the term *hypnosis*. It later became an accepted form of therapy as psychiatrists like Sigmund Freud popularized the concept by famously making it part of his practice and therapy.

Reports of "Past Life Memories" have been around for quite a bit as well. Mentioned in the Upanishads from ancient India, reincarnation is accepted in various forms by a number of religions from Hindus to Buddhists, the Taoists of China, American Native tribes, Aboriginal tribes of Australia to the Celts of England who all believed souls are immortal and after a fixed number of years after death, enter another human body. In the Middle Ages, there were a number or reincarnationist movements in Europe. The Cathars were considered such heretics by the Catholics that they sent them on to their next lives with great dispatch.

Over the centuries, a number of American thinkers embraced the concept, including Benjamin Franklin, Mark Twain, Walt Whitman, General George Patton and Henry Ford who said "I adopted the theory of reincarnation when I was 26. Genius is experience; some seem to think it is a gift or talent, but it is the fruit of a long experience in *many* lives."

According to the Pew Research Center survey, one out of four Americans believes in reincarnation. But aside from being a belief system relegated to religious dogma, it didn't begin to be examined by Western science until the 1950's when hypnosis and past life regression became a form of therapy in the mental health field. It was new therapy, however, and during hypnosis a patient might be encouraged to remember things that didn't actually occur, and for this reason, many considered the role of the psychiatrist's leading questions the culprit in supposed past life memories. That led the scientific community to believe these memories were the result of "Cryptomnesia," narratives created by the subconscious mind, using imagination, forgotten information and suggestions from the therapist; in other words, entirely made up.

In terms of popular culture, the first widely reported case of a remembered past life in the U.S. was that of an American woman in the 1950's who remembered details of a life lived in 19th century Ireland by a woman named Bridey Murphy. Research at the time could not verify her story and eventually her saga fell into disrepute. Past life regression and hypnosis became a common joke on television shows, from Lucille Ball getting hypnotized into becoming a criminal on "I Love Lucy" to Albert Brooks' "Defending Your Life" about a patient who has a peer life review with hilarious consequences.

---

[3] Wikipedia; Hypnosis, en.wikipedia.org/wiki/Avicenna

Dr. Ian Stevenson of the University of Virginia took up the subject of reincarnation as a serious topic in the 1970's and with the benefit of research, time and money, over 30 years was able to catalogue numerous cases that proved, from a scientific point of view, that reincarnation could at least be categorized and studied. Stevenson said he was skeptical of past life memories during hypnosis because like most critics, he feared the therapist could or would interject false memories via the questions.[4] However, Dr. Brian Weiss, a Yale trained psychiatrist, encountered spontaneous past life regressions in his work and turned those revelations into his bestselling book "Many Lives, Many Masters."

Recently the New York Times noted that "Past life regression" has returned as an acceptable tool for many psychiatrists.[5] A number of hypnotherapists, including those interviewed in this book, recount patients spontaneously going into a past life regression during a session, and being cured of their psychosomatic illness after examining the source of their illness or pain. There isn't a known medical reason behind these spontaneous cures, other than "the placebo effect." As we'll learn in this book, there may be other verifiable origins involved.

Dr. Michael Newton had a similar experience as Brian Weiss. A patient spontaneously regressed into a previous life, and despite being skeptical about past life regression in general, Newton was able to verify that a British soldier had lived and died as described during his session. As a result, Newton began doing past life regressions, and as he as put it "was dragged kicking and screaming into the movement."

Over the following decade, Newton began quietly cataloguing his cases of patients who could remember past lives. One day his focus took a giant leap forward. A client under hypnosis described the "life between lives," where everyone reportedly goes after they die and, with the help of their soul mates, decide how and where they'll return. Newton began to research this new field more fully with his patients, and after 20 years of intense research, published his first of four books in 1994.

Looking a bit like Charlton Heston, Newton, late 70's, has an easy, laid back manner. Having retired from his practice as well as stepping aside from his full time duties with the "Newton Institute," he's weary of fighting the battles with those who feel his research attacks their belief systems. However his pale blue eyes still flash when he talks of debating critics.

---

[4] "A large part of what emerges under hypnosis is pure fantasy. Some of these "previous lives" have been traced back to historical novels." Interview with Omni Magazine, 1988.

[5] "Interest In Reincarnation is Growing," by Lisa Miller. NY Times 8-29-2010

INTERVIEW WITH DR. MICHAEL NEWTON

RM: Is hypnosis a valid scientific tool?
Dr. Michael Newton. A lot of people don't feel it is. Hypnosis is a study of human behavior, adequate scientific proof depends on your willingness to accept self-reports from the mind as data. When someone is in deep hypnosis, it's not something that can be programmed. Under hypnosis, people are very aware of who they are and have great insight into what they're telling you. Over thousands of cases there was consistency of reporting; it didn't matter whether a client had a deep religious belief system or not; once we had them in deep hypnosis, they all told us the same things.

What was your first past life regression?
I began practicing in 1956, a traditional psychotherapist using hypnosis to try to uncover childhood emotional and physical trauma. It was the year of the famous Bridey Murphy case - the Colorado housewife who remembered a previous life in Ireland. I'd get calls, "May I come for a past life regression?" I'd say "No, I'm traditional, not involved with "new age" thinking." I was very naive, really.

But then a client asked if I could see him about pain he was feeling in his side. He'd been troubled since childhood, and doctors said it was psychosomatic - they'd done x-rays and could find no physical symptoms. They told him he should see a psychiatrist. When he came, I couldn't find any earthly origins at all, so I gave him the command "Go to the origin of this pain."

Well, he jumped into the life of a soldier in World War I, when he was a British Sergeant and was being bayoneted. I couldn't believe it; this fellow was lying on the couch groaning while I was more interested in verifying if it was real – asking him the British unit he claimed to be with and a number of other facts - instead of desensitizing this horrible trauma he was going through. Eventually I did do that.

He called a few days later to say "There's no more pain, thank you." Well that didn't satisfy me, so I contacted the British war office and the Imperial Museum in London to find out if this British Sergeant ever existed and sure enough he died in 1916. From that case, I began taking past life clients. So I came kicking and screaming into this movement.

Sometime later, a woman came to me, depressed over having no friends and couldn't seem to connect with anybody. I reached a point of frustration when I couldn't seem to find any help, so I said "Go to the origin of your loneliness, especially if there's a group of people around you." I didn't know it, but "group" was a trigger word, because we exist between lives in soul groups - "cluster groups" we call them. Her face lit up. She got tears in her eyes and pointed to my office wall and said "I see them all."

I was thinking *Is she seeing them in this life? In a past life?* "Where are we?" I asked. "Oh," she said, "We're in the spirit world. I'm seeing all my soul companions, they're wonderful," and she began describing them. I probed more, took a lot of notes, and had a recording of the session. I found none of her soul companions in her life today and she was lonely because of it. After she left, I said to myself *This can't be happening to me.*

I'm the world's worst cynic, skeptic, and past lives was enough of a jolt of cold water, and now this? I studied my notes and the tape for a long time, and then with other clients, I began exploring it more and more. Once I started, I couldn't stop. I closed my practice to all other forms of hypnotherapy and worked quietly and alone. I didn't go to hypnosis conferences, I didn't want to read metaphysical books, and I just wanted to do the research by myself. After twenty years I realized I *should* write a book, so I began collecting better case notes with an eye to writing "Journey of Souls."

What was the reaction from colleagues or your wife when you came home with this information?

Frankly I didn't go public until the first book was published. I had a lot of criticism from my colleagues; "How dare you keep this information from us, you didn't get our input." I said "I did not want to be influenced by your thoughts; I didn't want to introduce bias into my work."

My wife is a nurse trained in psychology, and she was, like myself; initially skeptical. I had to talk to somebody, and what better person than my soul mate, who didn't tell her friends, but quietly absorbed all this. Eventually she came to really believe in what I was doing.

A TYPICAL SESSION

Can you walk us through a typical Life between Life session?
People come in because there may be a relative who recently died, or emotional trauma from losing a child. This work is not to supplant therapy they should receive from a licensed trained professional; it's intended to provide them with answers about their inner being. One of the things clients don't understand until they experience it is that there is a dual nature to all of us. We have our brain ego if you will, and we have a soul ego, and when they are combined it creates one personality and one lifetime.

The first hour we pick a couple of childhood memories to get a sense of them recalling events earlier in this life, to prepare them to answer questions on a deeper level. Then we take them into their most immediate past life, because it's their most recent experience. It's very brief as it's not intended to be a discourse on past lives. There are a number of past life therapists that don't have a clue about Life between Lives therapies - they think it's grayish 'limbo' that has no significance. But we then cross from the death experience into the spirit world, into the afterlife; it's an interesting and exciting time for the client because they begin to really see their soul.

Friends, relatives or their spirit guide, usually both, come to greet them - when a client sees their immortal teacher for the first time they're usually blown out of their minds. Some religious people think they see Jesus or Buddha or Mohammad coming towards them but they quickly realize, "Oh, no, no, no... this is my personal teacher who's been with me since I was created as a soul."

From there, we move to interesting aspects of the spirit world, perhaps soul groups which range from 3 to 25 souls, the average client has about 15. These are all friends, relatives, spouses, dear friends in this life and some clients are shocked by who's there. There are other soul groups, nearby affiliated souls, that may play an important part in certain lives. There are reasons for that, and we try to explore it.

From there, they typically go in front of a group of wise beings - some call them "The Elders" or "The Wisdom Makers" - wise beings who are a step or two above their guides. These are non-incarnating beings, they're about as close to God as we get, and there's usually a very interesting discourse. They may ask the patient "How do you think you did in your last life?" They're very gentle people.

An interesting thing happens when they're ready to return in the next incarnation; there's a life and body selection library where people choose different kinds of bodies and who they think they can work best with. Their elders and guides have a hand in their selection before they come forward into the next life. It's a fascinating process. What's key is there's such order and discipline there and yet it's a very compassionate loving relationship. It isn't one that involves the kinds of things we see on Earth with a hierarchy of beings who lord over you and engender fear. There is infinite forgiveness and understanding there. We all make mistakes, some of them terrible, and that's all forgiven once we cross over.

When the clients wake up after one of these long sessions, some of them are crying and some of them are laughing, some of them can't talk - and generally there's just this "Wow. I can't believe it." Trying to process what's happened.

AFTERLIFE CLASSROOMS AND THE COUNCIL OF ELDERS

I've spoken with a few people who've referred to their own recurring dreams of being in a classroom somewhere in the Universe, some working with or without energy. Also, I'd like to know more about "The Elders."

We get flashbacks from time to time that break through that amnesiac block, folks who've had no LBL experiences, and just ordinary people that don't know about our work. Suddenly they're in a classroom in their dreams and they think "Hmm. That's a strange image; where's that coming from?" Most of us between lives spend time in a spiritual classroom. They are usually described as buildings, a library, or the place where they meet their council looks like a beautiful domed structure and in some cases a temple. Of course, there aren't buildings in the ethereal space between lives, but people free-associate or have flashbacks of buildings; "I'm in a classroom, I have people around me that I know, there's a teacher..."

Essentially we're given instruction by a Specialist Soul in areas we may have a talent or affinity for. They may be areas we'll specialize in after our incarnations are over - when we will be helping others. I often hear about an energy creating class where they're working with raw energy to create certain things.[6] I have the theory a lot of what we see on Earth in terms of plants and animals and geographics has been created by groups of advanced souls.

When we visit the Elders, we talk about our lessons and what we might do differently in the future. We're not standing before God or a Creator or a Source - But people describe feeling kind of a God like presence at these meetings. It's hard for people to describe it; I need to speak to someone who's not incarnating anymore to give me answers to that sort of thing. Once in a while I got a highly advanced client who was in their last series of incarnations, who'd open the door a little bit, and it's beautiful to listen to.

What kinds of questions would you like to know the answers to from this work?

When I get an advanced client in my chair, I feel sorry for them because I'm a relentless inquisitor. I've asked the question "What does it all mean?" with certain advanced clients. One thing I've learned is that we are only one of many universes. I've been able to hear about nine or ten dimensions, either parallel universes or universes that overlap in timelines, through patients. Once you leave Earth, of course, you're not in linear time anymore, you're in what we call 'now time'[7] - which is past, present and future... that's the best I can do on the question about creation - I wish I could tell you more.

QUANTUM PHYSICS AND THE AFTERLIFE

What do you think about the concept that photographs may be captured time?
It feeds into what we know about quantum physics - the Cherokee Indians believe no event in time is ever lost. I think from what I have discovered, *nothing is ever lost*; every moment of time represents particles of energy. It's like a movie that's being shown. That frame is there forever and can be recalled in the spirit world. Souls are able to go back to any event in any past life and review it completely.

This is one of things we do that is so valuable. When they're in the spirit world, in a library or a classroom, they're able to recall everything from their past; nothing ever dies and when you have past, present and future all conjoined into "now time" think of the advantage that brings to studying and reviewing what you've done and how you can make it better.

---

[6] These energy classes are mentioned in a number of sessions in this book.

[7] For those who watched the final episode of "Lost," one of the characters refers to "Now time" as the reason they all had multiple time lines.

There are possibilities and probabilities in the time continuum and there have been wonderful books about parallel universes, the "Holographic Universe" by Michael Talbot for example. It's very much in synch with reports we get from clients who've never read the books, so I feel the knowledge we're gaining now is greater than it's ever been about our inner being and the forces behind our creation.

Why hasn't this information been available earlier in our history?
I think there are a couple of reasons. We've never been so over-populated in history, with so many of us running in so many directions. Second, I think it's the pervasive use of drugs which has even reached our elementary schools - when someone is taking drugs to "escape from reality" it shuts down the soul. And maybe the powers that be decided it's time to loosen up this amnesia bloc we all have when we come into this world so we're able to gain information that perhaps earlier was not really available."

INTERVIEW WITH PEGGY NEWTON

I spoke with Dr. Newton's wife, Peggy. Michael told me his entire life he'd had a vision of meeting a woman dressed in a white uniform named Peggy. After he came out of the service, he saw an ad in a magazine that reminded him of his lifelong vision. A poor grad student on the G.I. Bill, he caught a bus and asked the driver to "Let me know when we are near the largest hospital in Phoenix." The driver let him off next to a dormitory, which was fortuitous as he thought it was the main entrance. When he walked inside and asked "Do you have a nurse named Peggy?" a woman brought her out to meet him. He knew the moment he saw her she was the woman in his dreams, and they've been together ever since.

RM: How did you meet Michael?
Peggy Newton: I was a student nurse and he was in graduate school. He had this feeling about a woman with dark hair dressed in white he was supposed to meet named Peggy. Off he went looking for a dark haired Peggy in a white uniform; he maintains from the moment we met he knew I was going to be with him for this life. And had probably been with him for many lives.

Can you remember that day?
He came to our dorm and we had a charming house mother on duty. He said "I can't remember her last name but I'm looking for a Peggy with dark hair." Then he told me this rather crazy story I won't repeat, because it made no sense to me at the time, when I asked him to sit down and clarify why he was there. We wound up talking for four hours; I went upstairs and told my roommates I'd met the man I was going to marry. We've been married almost 51 years.

What was it like when he first came home to tell you about a past life regression?
I thought it was too bizarre. "Past lives?" I had my medical scientific brain and I tended to put that to one side. I did think he might be 'over the bend' though, and worried about his sanity. But then he played me the tapes. His clients' tapes are private, so anything I heard never left me, but I realized these people were all saying the same things about the spirit world. Seeing the same things, saying the same things, how could that be if it wasn't true? You just can't take strangers through an experience where they relate stories that are all the same. I became a real believer at that point, and then I became a true fan."

I felt it key to hear from his wife that she'd been hearing the tapes of his sessions dating back to the beginning of his research. She confirmed the detail her husband had avoided metaphysical sections of bookstores during his research so he wasn't be influenced by other's work in the area. Newton said he'd had over 7000 patients who said the same things about the hereafter while under deep hypnosis. If true, then Michael Newton's work may become one of the greatest discoveries in human history.

My documentary on reincarnation took a turn after this interview. I began to focus on the science behind reincarnation, as well as stories of people who either had a direct experience of remembering the life between lives, or those who've spontaneously gone there via near death experiences or other means. I began with interviews with hypnotherapists trained by Newton as well as others who'd never heard of him. I also filmed sessions with various patients, some friends of mine who were skeptical about the entire process, and finally, I was invited to have my own session which I would film as well.

As a matter of logic, either what these patients were saying about the afterlife was true, or it wasn't. If it was true, then others must be able to visit the same place without his help or guidance. Also, if it was true, then there must be cases of others who've traveled this same route, without the direct guidance of Michael Newton. I was invited to film a session conducted by a Newton trained hypnotherapist, Paul Aurand. I was about to head *down the rabbit hole.*

"I know I am deathless. No doubt I have died myself ten thousand times before. I laugh at what you call dissolution, and I know the amplitude of time."

- Walt Whitman

CHAPTER 3
HUMANITY IN THE HOLOCAUST

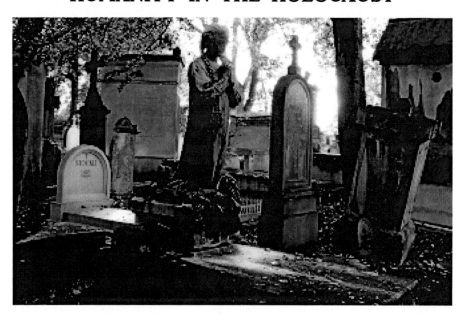

"In Italy, the country where fascism was born, we have a particular relation with the Holocaust, but as a turning point in history, it belongs to everybody in the world. It is part of humanity."

- Roberto Benigni

At the training session for the Newton Institute, I was ushered into a large hotel meeting room, where I was introduced to a room full of hypnotherapists on hand to watch a demonstration. "Noreen,"[8] one of the fellow candidates agreed to be filmed doing a session for fellow students. She's a successful hypnotherapist herself, has helped many people with past life regressions and life between life sessions, and after her session, I asked her a number of questions; she said she was unaware of this particular past life before this session, and had no inkling it was part of her spiritual background.

Since retired, Dr. Newton attended the conference in an advisory role, sitting off to the side to make notes on a large white board during the session to clarify what the students were observing. While Noreen reclined on a large divan in the center of the room, President of the Institute, Paul Aurand conducted the session. I put my camera on a tripod and settled in; not knowing that in three hours, everything I knew about the planet would go through a paradigm shift.

NOREEN'S JOURNEY WITHIN

(Paul spent 20 minute of regression techniques to take her back through her life).

Paul: Let's go further in time along your lifetime, back to one of your very earliest, first memories. A pleasurable one. Five... four... three... two... one... be there now.
I'm in my crib and I'm able to hold onto the side and move my legs up and down. It's nap time but I'm not tired. There's a piece of wallpaper that catches my attention and I start peeling it off. I'm kind of fascinated to see how that's unraveling.

How's it feel there?
I'm curious about everything. I want to get out of the crib.

Do you try?
I throw my leg over the top and climb down; it's not too well received. My mother wants me to take a nap so she can rest and have some time alone. She's not happy about the wall paper.

Allow yourself to go even deeper. Rise up from that scene and travel back further, go back to that special time in the womb, after conception and before birth... three, two, one.. Be there now.
It's pretty dark. I'm excited to be in this little baby body, there's a lot to do, but my mom is tense.

NOTE: Part of this method is to ask the patient what they remember about the womb. To my surprise, people always have an answer that isn't "How could I possibly know?" The answers generally speak of being constrained, constricted, or feeling otherwise cramped, but always relate to their primal connecting to their

---

[8] Not her real name, and where necessary, I've substituted pseudonyms for people's real names.

mother. Many speak of "trying to calm" their mothers, or "sending waves of love" to them.

THE SPIRIT JOINS WITH THE BABY

How do you sense that?
Through tension in her muscles and uterus and I'm trying to help her relax by pushing and moving, but that seems to make it worse and she's scared too. I feel it in my body, I respond to the fear and the nervousness, the anxiety. It goes through me like a wave. I think she doesn't feel prepared at all.

You work to try to soothe or calm your mom?
I think if I move she might connect with me and it might help her to relax, but she doesn't respond the way I'd like her to; she gets more tense. So I stop moving so much and just try and send her love.

How do you send her love?
I have a thought of love and I merge it with the sensation of what it feels like to me – love – and then let it radiate outwards.

What's your sense of why you're coming here?
I'm coming for my mother because she has difficulty loving herself. It translates into anger at times, which she later directs towards me and my siblings. I'm supposed to teach her how to love herself and love others by simply loving and accepting her. But that isn't always easy for me either.

Can you help me understand that a little better?
(Sighs.) I often pick challenging situations to incarnate in. It's not that I haven't been with loving families, but it seems this is part of what I do; go into families that need to feel love.

Do you spend all or most of your time in this body being ready to be born?
Not initially. Towards the end.

Initially, let me know where you go or what you do outside of the womb.
I go with my guide and we work on how to create love and hold onto it while in the body. I like to be with the baby too, I come back happily to move the body, to remember how that feels.

When do you fully join with the fetus?
Around 7 and half months.
    NOTE: It's also part of the methodology to ask a client when they joined the fetus from the spirit world. According to Michael Newton's research, souls, or spirit energy, don't join the human body until after the fourth month (reportedly

for physiological reasons). All births are part of an agreement, or shared communion, between the spirit energy and the human body. Accordingly, no one is born without a spirit, and a fetus that doesn't come to term due to miscarriage (or abortion), may have planned the event in advance in order to help the parents' spiritual progression. There are cases in the research where the spirit stays after the miscarriage, and is born later, or through a close relative.[9]

LIFE AND DEATH DURING THE HOLOCAUST

All right, take a nice breath, even deeper. Let's continue on our journey… travelling through a tunnel of light… Three, two, one, and be there now.
It's very bright out.

What's happening?
It's a heavy feeling. (Sighs) People are dying around me.

What are you doing?
We're being rounded up. And uh… we're in a camp. (Cries)

Remember you can hover above if you want.
People are dying because they're hungry. Some are taken away and they don't come back and we don't know what's happened to them. All kinds of rumors are abounding about what's happening. I'm an older woman; I have brown hair, but it's graying.

Who rounded you up?
Soldiers, officials of the government have rounded us up. And we were in this horrible place.

Help me understand where this is.
It's somewhere in the 1940's. This is very disturbing. We're all afraid. The sense is that we're clinging onto hope that somehow we'll survive this, but there's a sense that we won't survive this.

Let's move back in time a bit, how did you come to be in this place?
We heard rumors. We know that our people were disappearing.

Help me understand who "our people" are.
The Jewish people. We were living in fear but we thought if we just became invisible and passive that everything would be alright, this would pass. And of course getting closer to God, getting closer to our faith, there would be some protection there.

---

[9]   Carol Bowman "Children's Past Lives: How Past Life Memories Affect Your Child"

Now help me to understand who 'we' is. Is there a family? Do you have children? A spouse?
Yes. I have a husband, I have adult children. I have a daughter and a son, and between my son and daughter, I have five grandchildren. I love them very much.

Do you recognize any of them in your current life?
My grandson is my youngest son in my life now.

And there… what's his name?
There his name is Jacob.

And what's your relationship with your grandson Jacob?
I love him so much. I have so much hope for him, so much promise for him; he's such a sweet, loving, bright child...

So we're going to move forward to the end of this life, so we can move past this and work on this in a little bit, is that all right?
Mm-hm.

Moving to the end, you've done this many times before. Tell me how that life comes to an end.
I've been separated from all my family, from my children, from my grandchildren. And I don't know what's happened to them, so I'm hoping somehow they're all right, but my sense is - they're not. And we're told, a group of us, we're going to take showers and we all know that we're not.

I mean, we hope we're going to be moved to a more comfortable place and have food, and there's part of me that wants to scream and fight, there's another that says just stay small, stay connected, and remember that love is what really matters.

And so we go… into the place where the showers are, and there is such a funny smell all the time… The odor is uh, we smell it at other times too.

Before we go in, just tell me what your name is?
Anna Pachinski.[10]

So moving quickly, into the showers, notice where you are. What happens?
It's over pretty quickly. We're gathered together and we press against each other. There's a commotion and I'm just trying to stay calm. I take deep breaths so it can be over faster, and then it's done.

Are you moving away from the body now?
Yes. Pulling away. I'm looking upwards...

---

[10] Doing research online through a database that tracks victims of the Holocaust, I was able to find an Ana Pachinsky, as well as Anna Pashinsky, and Yakob Pietszyunski as names of people from Warsaw who died in the Holocaust. (This interview is used with permission from SoulTherapies.com)

What do you see?
It's dark at first, there seems to be lights all around me. I'm moving very, very quickly and I sense the presence of my guide near me. He's just there to encourage me, I guess, I'm excited about returning home, definitely about leaving that life behind.

How's it feel to be home?
It feels really good.

How are you greeted?
I'm enveloped by loving arms by my guide.

NOTE: Noreen was following the same path Michael Newton's patients followed in their sessions. She was taken through her previous life then asked to describe the manner of death from her past life. From there, it's an easier path to journey to the life between lives realm, where everyone reports being greeted by a spirit guide, or guardian angel if you will. This person is someone the client recognizes as having been their spirit guide for millennia. Noreen's description of these events follows the pattern of everyone I interviewed.

NOREEN'S SPIRIT GUIDE

Upon greeting you, what is your guide conveying to you in this welcome back?
There's some energy exchange between us. I respond very quickly, which is surprising. I'm just so happy to be home and it's like taking off this heavy cloak. I'm enjoying the presence of being back in this loving realm and his loving energy. He's encouraging me because I had the feeling I could have done better in that life - and he's just telling me I did good and not to second guess.

So just take that into the depths, that you did well.
I'm telling him I wished I could have saved those around me and he's telling me that wasn't my job, that wasn't what I was there to do.

And what does he say your job was?
He says my job was to love those souls in my life no matter how short it was. To be open and loving and supportive and caring and encouraging and to that extent I did a good job. I wasn't supposed to save their lives, and my family felt my love and my friends did as well.

What age were you when that life came to an end?
47.

So you had a sense of wishing you could have been of more assistance?
He's very clear that's not what we planned or agreed to. It was just to be loving, to

embrace my family and friends and community. I did feel fear and anxiety but was always able to come back to a very peaceful place pretty quickly.

Is this something you've been working on?
I've been working on this for a number of lifetimes; being a loving presence in my own existence and in the lives of others.

Do you have a question for your guide?
We're going to another center.

Can you describe that to me?
It looks like a library, it has the stately serious kind of atmosphere, but this is more of a classroom we're going to. There are other students, other beings there and as we come in to the room, there is an instructor there.

   NOTE: Classrooms in this "Afterlife University," as we'll see, is a common sight. From my research, the classrooms usually have to do with energy transfer, healing practices, or the creation of objects with the use of energy.

CLASSROOMS IN THE AFTERLIFE

Can you describe this instructor to me?
He's a perfect blend of energies, a lot of masculine energy, but more of a balance. He has a very large presence and he appears more as light.

Have you worked with him before?
I have, and my spirit guide is his assistant to some extent.

The other students, are you familiar with them?
We do experiments together and it's interesting. We're a part of this group and we feel cohesive and we know each other; but it's a little bit more like comrades, partners, than students.

If you were going to give the group a name or purpose, what would it be?
We're not an advanced class; we do experiments working with energy. We're working with energy so we can create things.

What kind of things?
It's very basic working with molecules and atoms, and seeing if we can get them to take just elemental shapes or forms, if we can turn energy into a rock or a flower or a container, anything that we can slow down the energy and give it more substance.

You do this as a group?
We do both in a group and we partner up and work with each other and sometimes we work alone.

How many are you?
I'm seeing 20. I see that others are joining us too, sometimes there's less – they go other places or they go off with their guide or guides and do other activities, so that is not a fixed number, it's fluid.

So you've been away awhile.
I'm back. They greet me, although I get the sense I'm there even when I'm not there.

Even when you're on Earth?
Yes.

Are they able to benefit from what your experience is on Earth?
We benefit from all of our experiences. We don't benefit from one more than another; it's all an integral part of it.

Let's go deeper. Describe to me the energy you experience there.
There's excitement, a sense of responsibility, we take our work seriously, but there's humor too.

If we were to hold a mirror, so you could see your reflection, what color are you?
I look more like light.

I understand. What color is your spirit guide?
Royal blue. He has tinges of purple, violet. And there are some specks of other colors, iridescent specks that reflect truer colors, so he's sort of sparkling.

NOTE: At some point during his research, Dr. Newton asked a client "If I held up a mirror to you, what would I see?" and the client described various colors. Newton began to catalog them, coming to the conclusion that younger souls had lighter colors, and older ones had darker colors. As we'll see in these interviews, it's a common question about a soul's color, not to be confused with 'the color of a person's aura,' which is reportedly based on other factors.

RECONNECTING WITH THE ETERNAL SPIRIT

Take a breath and go deeper, knowing that what's really important is that you know and understand. Is there more there we need to do or explore in this group?
Only to say it's a lot of fun to be there, fun to actually create something. We can create some things with substance. They have physical properties that are very palpable and discernible, but we can also create vibrations, emotions and thoughts. It's fun to experiment with what humor can make, what love can make, what anger can make. We experiment with all of the possible emotions we're aware of and then we choose forms. Then we do some work with our energy field, to just create objects.

You can make tangible objects, but also work with emotions. Is there a common theme?
There are elements of working with imbuing physical things, objects, or form with love. There's also - this has application in healing too – some of what we're doing can be healing to others. Not everyone needs this, not all souls need this, but some do.

So you're working with love and healing energy?
The real theme is how do we put into physical form these higher vibrations? What's coming through now is the universe is comprised of a very high vibration and that vibration can be called love. But it's not personal love; it is a vibration that's very, very high, beyond... I can't even explain -- it's not romantic love, it's a love that respects and honors and sees the connection of all things.

Is this a love we're able to experience on the Earth plane?
Oh yes. When you feel it, it's very peaceful. There's a silence, a silence that is so pure. And when you are in that place, you absolutely know we are all connected - it's as if we are all flying sparks and we all connect to each other. It's beautiful. It's complete peace and love and there's no sound.

And this is something that you and your group are working with?
When you really see it, it's as if the universe has billions of lights and they all connect. You can't count them all and there's such stillness and wholeness there... and the heart, or what could be perceived as the heart, is so open and it's Love -- it's overwhelming.

Beautiful. Where does your guide take you next?
I'm asking if I can go somewhere to view past lives. He's taking me to a place we can do that.

Can you describe this place?
It's a formal building with pillars, white and an inscription between two pillars at the arch. My spirit guide is going with me; I'm interested in seeing a lifetime where I was close to a loving person.

    NOTE: In many sessions, people refer to a library where lifetimes are chosen. Reportedly, a soul returns to this area to see various possibilities they might choose from for future incarnations. The descriptions of the life selection area vary upon a person's ability to describe what they're seeing along with the powerful emotion associated with seeing past lives or mistakes.

BODIES OF LIGHT

Take the time you need to do a review of those lifetimes.
We're looking at where I originated from. My first awareness of existing as a separate being is in this place and we don't have bodies, we are more like light. We

have form, but not substance. It's sort of being like crystals. We don't have bodies but thoughts are very important there, because whatever you think happens. It's very important thoughts are pure. We don't have the need for special connections between people. We don't feel the need to have families; the souls that *are* there, are there. This body is nice because it's fluid in the movement. Not fluid like liquid, but transparent.

So if you don't procreate, how do you come into being?
It seems to me that our souls were just *there* in this place.

How would you describe this place?
Very light, soft colors.

Is there a predominant color?
More pastels but iridescent. And we work with thoughts to create other things. I'm trying to see or find out what it is we really do.

What is it that you're doing, learning or working on?
All of existence is holding vibration, but they're different vibrations and all really important. So the vibration we're holding has to do with a higher level of thoughts. And we can see exactly how quickly thoughts manifest into feelings, into physicality. And if we let our vibration lower and our thoughts lower, we have an opportunity to see what happens -- what's manifested by lowering the energy. Conversely if we keep our thoughts and vibrations high, we can see the full potential.

So you're really learning about this with others there?
Yes. I wish I could understand more.

Take your time with it and report to me in a bit.
This is what I'm seeing and sensing; at one particular time, we all came together. We were going to send a higher frequency into the surrounding spaces but somehow we didn't hold focus and then it became a mis-experiment. Our planet was destroyed. And while no soul perished, we became displaced, and that's a lonely feeling when you're displaced.

NOTE: Reportedly, not everyone has reincarnated on Earth, there are other galaxies, or planes of existence we can choose to go to. Also we weren't "hatched" at the same time, at the inception of the Universe, or the "Big Bang"- reportedly it's an ongoing process. Noreen's memory of a past life on another planet might not be a universal memory for everyone – we have these options of places to reincarnate, including other realms of existence. However, it certainly bears examination if only as an environmental warning to our own.

WHY WE CHOOSE OUR LIFETIME

What brought about the end of this planet, this mis-experiment you mentioned?
Somehow goals and objectives became personalized in people's minds. I think there was a touch of vanity and it tainted the work we were doing. Interesting how easy it was for it to become contaminated. Didn't take a whole lot.

How does all this relate to your current body and life on Earth?
How important it is to work together. To not allow oneself to feel greater than others. To feel a part of and connect with everyone and everything, and not go off on personal agendas. It's a collective and this dense reality here on Earth is an opportunity to play and experiment and feel and be. So it's going from one reality of not being in the physical to one that's in the physical.

In this other place, we thought because we didn't have bodies it was so much better. In retrospect, attachments can always be formed and there are always consequences. It's easier to see that working on Earth; it's more in our face. This is actually a wonderful opportunity to see how negative behavior hardens and crystallizes. But wherever you exist contains the opportunity to learn.

So now that your guide has reviewed this, original place of being, these experiments and this deeper purpose, are there other lifetimes that he wishes you to reveal?
There was a community I lived in a long time ago, that was love based and everyone was really joyful and happy, I often want to go back there, but I can't. But it was cheerful loving, supportive and happy. An easy life because everyone supported everyone else.

Was that here on Earth?
Yes.

So why did you and your guide choose to be here on Earth again?
To continue working on being within myself, and to help others find that in themselves. Because it's in everyone and everything, no matter what plane of existence they're in; it's in all of us.

What's there?
This place - of peace and love and joy and caring.

How much of your soul energy did you bring in this lifetime?
I feel it's 28%.

NOTE: We apparently agree to bring a certain level of energy into this lifetime. As we'll see in other interviews, this level of energy hovers between 25% to 50%. According to one hypnotherapist I interviewed, "If we brought all our energy to this human form, we'd blow the circuits." However, it does lead one to ask, "What's the other portion of our energy doing while we're here on Earth?" Do we have access to it? Could it be that religious icons in our history had more access to their energy? Through proper training, how can we access this energy? These concepts are explored in ensuing chapters.

THE AMOUNT OF ENERGY WE BRING WITH US TO THIS LIFE

Is that adequate? A good choice?
39% would have been more helpful, but I was wrong, I could have brought more.

You might ask if now would be the right time to visit those wise beings we know as the council. (Paul told me later that because of time constraints, he might ask a "leading" question to move the demonstration along). As you approach please describe where they will meet and work with you.
It's a formal setting. It's very stately and the floors are marbled. My council is sitting at a table, crescent shaped.

NOTE: The "Council of elders" or "the wise ones" is a phenomenon reported in every life between life session, averaging six to twelve non reincarnating elders on each council. Basically, it's a peer review done by elder souls for our benefit – with their help and guidance we get to benefit from their knowledge about our lives and how it relates to our overall spiritual progression. People make two trips to see their council, once upon our death, and once before the return to life to go over what lessons are to be learned.

A TRIP TO THE COUNCIL OF ELDERS

How many are there?
Seven. They seem more transparent than solid and there's an appearance of robes because of the fluidness they have. I see a beautiful royal blue color and light purple.

Is there one central figure?
There's one in the center that will serve in that role. My guide has gone over to stand by the council. I'm standing; I like to stand before them.

And what do you feel standing before them?
Gratitude. I feel honored and such great love coming from them, and of course, my love for them is almost overwhelming.

What are they communicating to you?
They're very supportive but I have some questions I want to ask. I'm addressing the main chair person, but it's addressed to all.

Does the response come from the chair person?
He filters the input he gets from everyone and when he speaks, he's speaking for all.

What do you ask?
How they think I'm doing in this present life. I also want input about the most recent one.

When you've done that let me know how they respond.
(Laughs) They say "Do you have to ask us the same question every time you come back?" They're tired of me being insecure when I get here; they're asking "What do *you* think?" As I stand before them, it seems like all of that becomes so unimportant because this message keeps coming -- from them and from my guide -- that everything I do and everything everybody else does is just fine, it's all part of the process. Whatever choices I make, they're perfectly fine choices and it's the reaction I have to the choices that creates a problem.

They're saying although some actions are more harmful or destructive, they cause a bigger reaction, and the reaction is important to observe because it's a teaching tool. What's important is once you learn the lesson, let it go and don't keep repeating it, because the more you do that, the more you attract the same in yourself. Just let it go.

Can you ask them about why it was necessary to go through this lifetime in the Holocaust?
The impressions are coming so fast, there's quite a few. One was to experience the importance of family, the love of family and community and to know that sometimes it doesn't go the way people want it to in the physical world. I just wanted to be with them but nothing is permanent.

Another reason was to practice being calm and centered and to conquer my fear. Fear is like a muscle and you can go through something so intense and not be afraid. I was working on that, and all of us collectively agreed to show the world something we needed to learn about hate, about greed, about anger.

Help me understand this.
All participants collectively showed others about love, greed, hate, love, strength, enduring no matter what; surviving the worst on a deeper level.

You mean those in the camps?
Those in the camps but also those that participated in them as well - the perpetrators. It was like there were many polarities being played out and all participants were a part of that demonstration.

So even the ones we would call the perpetrators had a role in this?
(A pause) You know from where I stand, I know this will sound really harsh, but it was much easier to be the victim than the perpetrator.

NOTE: At this point, my head shot up from my camera. *What did she just say? That it was harder to be a Nazi than a victim?* I'd never heard anything so politically incorrect in my life. For a moment I thought this had all been staged for the camera's benefit, the conference, the room, the session; then I realized I was viewing what she was saying through the lens of my experience. In order to hear what she was saying, I had to suspend my disbelief and really listen.

WHY WE CHOOSE A LIFE WITH DIFFICULTY

Don't judge it.
It was harder for the perpetrators because of the pain inflicted on a soul – even though everyone agreed, the pain of knowing you could cause such terrible hurt and suffering was unbearable for many of them. It also taught lessons in courage, learning about standing up for what was right.

That 'being invisible' you spoke of.
There were many of them that were invisible too. They were just going along because of their own fear and learning how much it hurts when we violate the laws we know to be true.

Are they speaking to you, or are they having you experience this in some way?
They're talking to me but I'm also experiencing it; they're showing me. As they're speaking to me, I see all the events going before me like a movie, and then I feel the feelings. I'm so familiar with what I felt in that body, I'm being given the opportunity to see and feel what the perpetrators felt -- I'm also seeing and feeling what victims were feeling, and if I were to put the two side by side, it sounds terrible, but I'm glad I was on the side of experience that I was on.

Because it was even more difficult to be on the other side?
Yes. Many of them have some corruption that will take healing, will take healing time. Because in order to be a part of this, they violated something their soul knew was wrong. They violated something in their own soul. Some were lured by it and fell down into it. Something inside got carried away; they didn't mean to be that driven to be destructive, but went beyond what had been planned. There are many lessons; heartlessness, not allowing ourselves to feel what others feel, shutting down and then becoming soulless in a sense. Then they were capable of anything; there was so much fear that if they opened up to what we were experiencing they too would be thrown in to the same circumstance. Others were afraid they would be engulfed with the horror and the pain of it all, and many of us on the other side closed our hearts too, the victims. Many lessons about the heart.

What a new perspective in learning. What more did they communicate to you?
That ultimately all souls are... I can't get the word that they're saying. They gave me an image of souls going into the hospital, ultimately the souls rehabilitate... There is no such thing as a throwaway soul. All souls have meaning and all souls have value and all souls have purpose and all souls are perfect. That it's a matter of finding our way back to that perfection after each lifetime on Earth. Specifically they're saying "Everything is as it should be, has purpose, meaning and value as to all the souls that participate."

What do they say to you about your soul's purpose?
They're telling me I'm one of the souls working towards being able to embody this. The part I saw in the classroom is about creating the synergistic energy of love and to acknowledge perfection in all things. Sending that message is very helpful to people as they continue on their path.

Perhaps you have something you'd like to ask them.
"How many lifetimes do I have to do on Earth?" (Laughs) They say "As many as you want; it's up to you." My impression is I'm coming back to continue the work I'm doing.

You mentioned they have deep blue robes. Anything else you notice?
I see a symbol in front of the chair person. It's virtual reality-like and it's spinning. It's gold in color and there are intertwining different lines, going up. It's almost as if it goes on forever, no end to it. It's a symbol for the interconnectedness of everything. I was able to go inside of it and it's beautiful; inside the center you are a part of everything, are in everything. When you're a part of everything, you are something grand; apart from it – you're nothing.

In a few moments we'll begin our return journey... and you'll be able to take some time to draw this symbol that helps you reconnect... fully awake by the count of ten."

As a filmmaker I feel I have an eagle eye for acting, writing or improvisation. But as I listened to the syntax, emotion and structure of her story, I couldn't find a hint of anything being made up, written or faked. She was as genuinely shocked by her story as I was. I went up to her after the session to retrieve the microphone while she was weeping over the revelations she'd encountered, saying she was overcome by the emotions she remembered from that life.

I asked if she'd ever remembered this particular lifetime before; she hadn't. I asked if she knew anyone who died in the Holocaust, or had any relatives who did so. She said she wasn't aware of anyone, and that was the first time she'd had any of those memories or experiences.

She said prior to the session, she'd asked Paul if it was possible to explore some tensions in her relationship with her mother, and also that her energy levels had been low as of late, and wanted to know if there was a way to change that. She said she was completely unprepared and shocked by her past life memory, but that it would help her with clients who'd experienced a similar tragedy.

"It was harder to play the role of a perpetrator than a victim in this lifetime." Was the implication being that some of the worst experiences that happen in humanity might have been created with our knowing participation? That the very things we find the hardest to deal with in our lifetime actually might be obstacles we willingly embrace so we can progress spiritually from them? That "stones in our path" may have been placed there with our tacit knowledge?

It was reminiscent of the supposed Gospel of Judas, the document recently found in Jerusalem where Judas claimed Jesus begged him to turn him over to the Romans. "But you will exceed all of them. For you will sacrifice the man that clothes me." He's saying "If you truly love me you will do this favor for me so I can fulfill my destiny." The idea a person might sacrifice their own happiness and well-being to benefit others strikes me as the height of compassion. That the golden rule; "Do unto others as you would have them do unto you," might include "in this lifetime."

After filming the session, my head was swimming. We're fully conscious between lives? We choose our parents and who we're going to return as? That we might return to lead difficult lives as an act of compassion? I interviewed Noreen to see if she had any motivation to make any of it up. I'm convinced, beyond a shadow of a doubt, she did not. I knew that filming more sessions would help me discover if the results could be duplicated. I next interviewed the hypnotherapist who conducted the session to see what he thought of her revelations.

"I am confident that there truly is such a thing as living again, that the living spring from the dead, and that the souls of the dead are in existence."

- Socrates

CHAPTER 4
ENLIGHTENMENT THROUGH ELECTRICITY

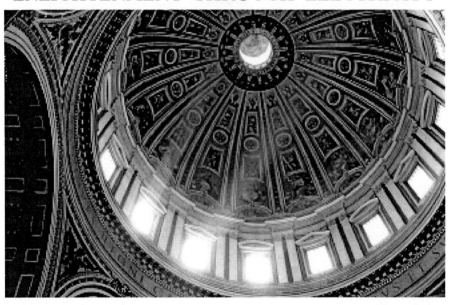

"We are born countless times; it is possible each being has been our parent at one time or another. Therefore it is likely all beings in the universe have familial connections."

- The 14ᵗʰ Dalai Lama

A funny, charming man with piercing blue eyes, Paul Aurand maintains an office in Manhattan and lives across the Hudson in New Jersey. A Master Hypnotherapist and Board Certified Medical Hypnotherapist, he's earned awards as "Therapist of the Year" and "Hypnotist of the Year." One of the first therapists trained by Michael Newton, he conducted the session for "Noreen."

RM: How did you come upon past life therapy?
Paul: One of my first experiences was with a young man in his 30's who had chronic sinus problems. He came to see me as a last resort, and while I was doing a regression with him – not past life, but 'regressing back to cause' - I took him to the origins of this chronic infection; he spontaneously regressed into a past life.

He described himself as a small child in Greece on a ledge, looking into this crystalline blue water that had something shiny down in it. He bent down to pick it up and fell into the water and drowned. And he began to drown in my office - he turned blue, he foamed, he scared me to death. I'd learned in my training if someone abreacted, to just take them through it, not shock them out of it, and after our session he said that he never had another sinus infection after that.

I'd read about past life regressions, but had never done one intentionally so I wasn't sure. I started to explore it a bit, and had another spontaneous past life regression with someone who came in with chronic shoulder pain. She was not a particularly spiritual person, she was a well-educated professor with chronic problems with her shoulder; she'd been diagnosed over a seven year period with bursitis, tendonitis, arthritis, and had been treated with physical therapy, cortisone injections, immobilization, physical therapy and now they were recommending exploratory surgery because they couldn't really resolve it otherwise. She felt healthy enough, but in pain - nothing else they'd done for her had really worked and she, sort of as a last resort, wanted to see if we could use hypnosis as a pain management technique.

So I used a standard technique called the "Burmese method," which is when you have a client focus on their pain and in their mind sort of make it bigger and then smaller to see if they can reduce the discomfort. And much to my surprise, she spontaneously regressed into a past life where she described herself as a slave with a small child who was starving. As she was trying to steal food for her child, she was caught by her master as she was stealing bread from the kitchen and she was beaten to death.

In the process of the beating, she was kicked in the shoulder, the area around her shoulder blade, and her shoulder was broken. I worked on just having her go through that process and we did a bit of helping her to release any residual pain there. And after the session, she reported that she had absolutely no pain in her shoulder. And I said, "Well, maybe you should make your appointment for next week," as she was used to doing with her other treatments, and when she came she was completely pain free. She very proudly told me she was back on the bowling team, something she loved to do, but hadn't been able to do for many years. I can't claim whether this is a valid past life memory for sure, but as long as it's therapeutic, as long as the patient benefits from it, I don't really care. It was with that attitude I began doing more intentional regressions into childhood, womb and past life.

A FLASH OF INSIGHT

How did you come to "life between life" therapy?
About 8 years ago I had a near death experience - I was struck by lightning. I had a number of residual issues; back pain, memory loss - about fifty million volts went through my body – and I was one of the lucky ones who survives that sort of thing. And about six months after, I had a regression session that took me back through the experience so I was able to release some of the trauma lodged in my body. In the session I remembered the near death experience and messages I received during the lightning strike. It was as a result of that, I began to explore how I could find a way to take someone into that profound near death experience, without actually having to get hit by the bus, or lightning, or whatever.

But it wasn't until I was called by Michael Newton to assist in his first training the light bulb went off - "This is it." This is how I can take someone into the spirit world, and explore their life's purpose, to review how they're doing, without having to have the physical body go through a death experience.

What do you remember about the lightning?
To my amazement, while I was being electrocuted, I had an awareness of what was happening. I had enough time to think, *I'm wearing rubber soled sandals*; there was this huge explosion, the loudest sound I've ever heard, and the jolt caused my entire body to convulse and threw me to the ground where I was out for a while. In the dead time, I experienced a couple of things which have stayed with me ever since. One is that we can have the concept or philosophy about unconditional love, but I don't think it's a common experience. I felt a complete reconnection with the whole, the "all being;" I was part of this universal sea of consciousness, if you will, I was "back home" and felt complete and unconditional love.

I later thought "How can I recreate that? How can I help someone have this between life experience and experience the same connectedness I did?" As someone goes back into spirit, as you heard during Noreen's session, some of the first words she spoke in the between lives were "I'm home." I think it's that longing for home and longing for love we as human beings carry with us through life. We look for it in our relationships and if we don't find it, we sometimes try to numb the pain we carry - it's there and it's always available, and I think this is a great avenue to get there.

A VISIT TO THE COUNCIL

Can you describe your own life between life session?
I was in a Civil War scene, I was in a pile of bodies, not quite dead yet. And then finally, I left that body and was met by my spirit guide, and pretty quickly was taken to this sort of domed place where the council, the wise beings were, and they were going to review my life with me.

As I approached this building, I thought I was going to go in and be judged. And one of the greeters came forward and said "There's no place for that here, this is not about being judged, there's no place for guilt or shame, that's not the way for you to enter here." I was reassured there need be no fear I was going to be judged.

Inside, I saw they had robes, I'd describe them as purely energetic and I felt that unconditional love again. They didn't really speak, but rather took me mentally through the experiences of a number of lifetimes. It wasn't like watching a movie or looking at them in a book - they actually put me into those lifetimes, so I could re-experience them from a different perspective.

One in particular was when I was a slave owner. I was by the side of the road and I was whipping my slaves. It was horrifying to see I could have that sort of attitude or mentality. I didn't even consider them to be human; I seemed to care more about my animals. It was very unpleasant. They showed me other lifetimes where I'd been callous about people's feelings.

Then the council brought me back and said "You're getting much better. The work you're doing now is benefiting people." They gave me the profound experience of reconnecting with the whole, being part of the Creator, part of the universe. An incredible feeling. Then they said "When you judge, when you criticize, when you discount, you separate - this is what causes the separation from the whole." They didn't talk about it as a philosophy, but gave me the experience of being separate again. "When you do this, you diminish the light for everyone." What a profound lesson for me and the world. We have learned from doing this work there are life lessons within each lifetime; we're here to accomplish certain things. It's a school where we learn and grow, but in addition to life lessons, there are soul lessons; lessons we may take many lifetimes to learn.

What do you think they meant by "diminish the light?" The energy in the Universe?
The life force; the light within us.

And they're saying that this happens whenever someone is negatively critical or judgmental? Gee, film critics must have a really hard time in the afterlife.

35

(Laughs). It seems to be a common theme. For example, in the regression of Noreen; here's someone who was in the Holocaust and was a victim, and as tragic and horrible as that is, from the perspective of the spirit world, from that expanded state of consciousness, she felt compassion for her perpetrators. She felt compassion for the pain the perpetrator's souls experience in playing that negative role. Not that it makes it right in any fashion, it is a terrible tragedy, it's horrible, and at the same time, things we judge from a human perspective as being right or wrong, or bad, may have a very essential role in helping others to help their souls progress.

SOULS WHO REMEMBER A LIFE WITH JESUS

Do you find that percentage wise, many of your clients died in World War II?
I've had quite a few people who in their regression are survivors of the Holocaust. I've had cases where there was a pattern of people who spoke about having once known a deep sense of being loved and loving, yet seemed to spend their lifetimes looking for it. Even though they found a loving relationship in this life, they were still experiencing a sense of disappointment, of feeling something was missing. Then, under hypnosis, they reconnect with it.

I've had a number of people go back to when Jesus was on the planet and being connected to his movement or experiencing life with Jesus or with those close to him; they had this deep sense of being loved. Then distraught when he was killed and living a number of lifetimes with the feeling "How could this have happened?" Some have said what a tremendous loss it was to humanity and "How could we exist without this sort of love?" and then not being able to find it anywhere on the planet.

And as they go into spirit, I remind them the energy isn't gone, it hasn't left the planet, love is still available, and they carry it within themselves. It's not out there with some other person or prophet or anyone else, it's within each of us. After spending a lifetime of relationships saying "How disappointing, what's missing?" to learn - not by a Priest or a Minister or Rabbi or Psychic or a Reader - but through their own inner experience during one of these sessions, that loving energy is *still* in existence and they carry it within themselves; what a profound relief for them. And they can offer it to others.

Some patients remember a past life with Jesus?
They remember a man who would tell stories, who would sometimes touch them, or his followers would touch them, and they would feel imbued with unconditional love. And they felt this huge loss when he was killed.

Do you ever encounter someone on the council wondering what you're doing in a session?
You generally allot four to five hours for a session and don't plan anything after because you need to rest. This was early in my career, I had a hypnotherapist coming in for a session, and I knew she'd go into hypnosis easily, so I only scheduled her

for two hours. Deep in the session she went to a place we call "soul groups," where we meet those souls we've often reincarnated with a number of times. There are usually around 6 or 8 souls, maybe 15 and they're often the primary group, and there's a secondary group loosely associated that's nearby.

I asked her how many were there, she said "Oh, about 100." Her Uncle came forward from this life who'd been a thorn in her side, humiliated her, shamed her, put her down; she was hoping not to meet him. He said, "Our contract, our agreement before this life was that you asked me to be a thorn because you wanted to work on your arrogance and your tendency to humiliate others. So I played that role, and man, that was really hard for me to do."

So here's this woman saying, "Wow, what a different perspective - he was someone I really hated and resented!" It wasn't something a therapist told her to work on, or a new age thought of "You should forgive him," but two souls learning from a very different perspective. The encounter took ten minutes alone. After each one came through and introduced themselves, I heard my next client arrive outside the door and thought, "Oh no, what am I going to do?" When the seventh soul came forward, he said "Tell him to stop rushing us." That was profoundly embarrassing; the first time I'd ever been addressed directly by someone through a client.

I've had three or four where the client was before the council, reviewing their life and the client said "The council wants to thank you for doing this work. They want you to know they need more humans to come before them, because this is really important work, they have messages they want to communicate. You're doing the work of reconnecting and please keep it up."

Finally, there was a fellow before his council and they gave him a message about something rather personal; that I was supposed to begin doing the work I'm doing now.

Any themes in the messages from the Great Beyond?
There are some universal messages that are simple, yet profound, usually about love and being loved. Noreen's question was "How can I feel the presence of my spirit guide more in my life and feel more connected?" His answer; "Meditate. Turn inward. Remember this occasion and you'll connect with me. I'm always with you. You are not alone." Many feel alone in the world, and the message is "You're not alone, your loved ones, guide, council - we're around."

Another theme is about judging negatively. Things we perceive as humans as bad or wrong - it's easy to say "Oh, he's a bad person," but when you look at the overall picture, those who play a negative role in your life may actually play an essential role. It's one thing to say from a religious perspective "You should forgive this person," but to see how that role may be essential, even if it appears to be negative, makes for a very different experience.

Someone can have a strong religious belief that doesn't include reincarnation, but when you take someone through one of these sessions, they have this mind boggling experience - it's a visceral experience on a soul and body level – they emerge *knowing* this to be true. It's far beyond a concept or belief. That's profound. One other common occurrence is a feeling of reconnecting to the whole. To know you and I are of the same essence makes it much more difficult for me to cause you harm, because it's harming me and the whole as well. That's a message for the entire planet; how we cause harm to others. It's more difficult to do knowing we are all the same. I'd love to see everyone have the opportunity to go through one of these sessions. It's wonderful that it's not a dogma, it's not a religion, but it's open to everyone.

Reincarnation, at least as I conceive it, does not nullify what we know about evolution and genetics. It suggests, however, that there may be two streams of evolution -- the biological one and a personal one -- and that during terrestrial lives these streams may interact.

- Ian Stevenson

CHAPTER 5
AQUAPHOBIA

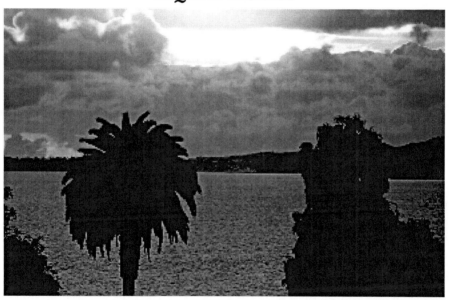

"If someone's phobia is eliminated instantly and permanently by the remembrance of an event from the past, it seems to make logical sense that that event must have happened."

- Dr. Edith Fiore

Where do phobias come from? Psychiatry, biology, genetics examine phobias that can be traced to misfiring in the brain – where an errant bit of electricity fires over a synapse and we find ourselves washing our hands incessantly, or hoarding items of comfort.[11] But is it possible some phobias come from before we were born?

This session was conducted at a Newton conference between *Peter Smith*, an Australian hypnotherapist with piercing blue eyes, and Sophia Kramer, an effervescent hypnotherapist from South Africa with an easy smile.

Peter: On the count of three I'm going to ask that you be there. One, two and three. Just be there now. Is it daytime or nighttime?
Sophia: Day. I'm outside

Do you sense that you're alone or with somebody else?
I'm not alone.

Allow me to know more. Look down at your feet.
Feet are bare. I'm five years old.

What's he wearing?
Bathing suit. Actually, I'm a little girl. I'm wearing just pants; it's too hot for a top.

I see. Know and understand this little girl and how she came to be there. Feeling safe and calm now. What name do you hear her father say?
It's on the beach in South Africa.

Is your daddy there? What does he call you?
My dad is there. He calls me "Mousy."

Is that what he calls you?
It's this lifetime. I almost drowned there.[12]

NOTE: After the session, I learned that Sophia had asked Peter to explore her terrible fear of swimming and being in the water. She'd had a recurring nightmare of being trapped in the water and swimming, but not getting anywhere.

FEAR OF DROWNING

Go back to the circumstances of that day. On the beach. Why are you there?
To play.

Who are you with?
My dad and my mom and my aunt and my cousin.

11 American Psychiatric Association. Healthyminds.org/Main-Topic/phobias.aspx
12 Later, Sophia said she was surprised that in her session, she went back to her own life as a little girl in South Africa, to the day that she nearly drowned in a lake.

Where do you live?
In South Africa.

If you asked her what year this was, what would she say?
1967.

Good, going deeper now. I want you to move forward in the day. What happens next?
I love the beach but I'm on this mattress and there are high waves.

Okay are you scared?
Yes.

I want you to feel safe; everything is going to be okay. Move forward in time.
Forward... (Begins to sigh heavily)

Go back to that time on the raft, when you were feeling anxious. Can you go back there?
Yeah.

Where do you feel that feeling in your body?
In my throat, and my ears and my throat, because this wave went over me and I gargled in the wave. (Coughs)

You're safe and secure. Take that beautiful bubble of light and drift up and out of the timeline, further back in time to the source of this feeling. Taking it to a deeper level.
    NOTE: As Peter spoke, Sophia's demeanor changed. Her face became agitated, stressed. She started to cough and choke, as if drowning. For a moment, I thought Peter might have to end the session. As it turned out, trained in abreaction, he was able to help her through this difficult memory.
    (She starts to cry). (Coughs)

Are you in another place? What name are you known in this place?
Hans.

Hans, what's happening right now?
(Coughs) I'm on this ring drifting in this cold water, and this huge ship above and I'm drowning.

What year is this? Allow yourself to know.
I hear "1872."

Everything's going to be okay, we'll look after you. Can you still see the boat?
A big ship. I was working on the ship.

Do they know you've fallen overboard?
Yeah. (Chokes, gasps)

Move forward in time. Move to when the soul leaves the body, through and past it.
(Coughs, chokes, gasps) I'm so angry! (Chokes, heavy breathing)

Move through until you are at peace. Feel your consciousness start to expand, feel the relief as your soul is free. Be there now. Feel the physical discomfort dissolving.
(Gasps, breathes easier).

Where are you Hans?
Floating above.

Do you feel at peace?
Yeah, but I'm still angry at that man watching it.

I want to know the circumstances that brought you to this place. You were working on the ship?
Yeah.

What role do you have on that ship?
Shoveling the coals in the heating room.

Have you worked on the ship for long?
(Nods). 12 years.

How old are you?
Just 35.

Hans, think carefully, recall the name of your ship. See yourself looking up at the ship, what's the first letter do you think?
I start to think why I'm Hans, when it's Irish. The ship is Irish. I think. Yeah. When I was on the dock I was in Ireland.

What about the name of the ship? What are you sensing? See the name on the side of the ship.
Lands.. M A N. I think.. Double N. Landsmann.[13]

Do you have a family?
I only have my mother.

---

[13] S.S. Lahns is the closest ship I could find; Landsmann is a nautical term for men who shoveled coal.

What country were you born in, Hans?
It was Denmark I think, but now it's not anymore. Now it's Germany.[14] I have a strong connection and I still feel Ireland, but the name of the ship doesn't match. I was born in Ireland and went on that ship in Denmark which is now Germany. It's all the same, they changed the border. And it was just for the ship - I love Ireland. (Smiles) My mom is Irish; she's an old Irish woman.

What city does your mother live in? See her now.
It's the middle of the Ireland. It is Newburg[15] or something. I love my sheep and fields of green.

Tell me; is your father still alive?
No. (Laughs.) Like all the Irish. Drank too much. Me too.

SOPHIA DISCOVERS WHO THE KILLER REALLY IS

I want you to return to the place where you passed over. After you've passed, all the physical discomfort has gone. Tell me, the person that you were angry at, why were you angry at them?
   He watched me drowning.

Did he not do anything?
Took pleasure in it.

I can understand that would make you angry. Why did he take pleasure in it? Was there something between the two of you?
When I go down there (to Earth) I don't see it, but up here I know it..

When you passed, you know more.
We shook hands before, I mean we made a contract, I just saw that we shook hands before that life, so it had a reason; I didn't see that before.

There was something for you to learn from this man in this lifetime?
Yes, we planned that. (For him to push me off the boat) Oh. He says "It was so difficult to do that to you."
   NOTE: This is a recurring theme, people who've agreed to perform a difficult task in your lifetime at your request. In this case, drowning someone you love.

Do you know this man?
Yes, I know who he is.

---

[14] The Southern part of Denmark was German from 1848-1917
[15] There is a Newborough,(pronounced Newburg) mid-Ireland. Sophia confirmed she'd not heard of it.

Do you understand that Mousy carried some fear of water in her body?
Yes.

And when we look deeper into that fear of water, do you sense there's a connection?
Yes. There's a thread. In this lifetime he didn't watch me drown, in this lifetime he saved me. (Cries) When I was a little girl on that raft, he was the one who saved me.

Was this man your father in another lifetime?
(Crying) Yes.

See him before you now, take his hand, and look into his eyes; are you ready to forgive him?
Oh yes. I see our hearts and everything is merging and it is just beautiful. And I see it all had a reason and I didn't make the connection before. But I still would like to understand why I had to have that lesson as Hans... I see. We had the contract so that I could learn a character flaw that I had to overcome and see what it felt like.

Are you ready to move further away?
Yes.

NOTE: In a few moments, Sophia saw the Captain of the ship who killed her, then realized that this same Captain is her father in her current life, and turns out to be the one who saved her from drowning when she was a little girl. (Something she wasn't aware of until this very moment.)

SOPHIA MEETS HER SPIRIT GUIDE

Go further into that beautiful soul state.
It's like the Milky Way, a hundred fold... And I'm a shooting star, shooting up.

Continue on your way. Let me know when you've reached your destination. Where are you now?
There are so many... (Sighs) There are so many. It's my main guide in front of all of them.

Ask him about the lessons. Is he male or female?
He has a male energy - But it's both... It's more male.

Ask him about your lesson as Hans. And report back to me in your own words.
Oh. I see. I was backstabbing people and I caused a lot of disharmony. And that was the contract.

Go down deeper now into this soul memory. Go down deeper now. Allow yourself to know the answer. Tell me more about the contract.

I see it like a movie - I see myself back shoveling these coals, I did something down there, it feels like... Oh. We had a problem with the ship and we hardly had any food left and we had to portion out the food, you know, they gave us each a portion. And I was... I was not honest, I was stealing from my comrades, and I just cared about myself to stay alive and others were dying... I was not a good person.

How do you feel about that lifetime?

I feel that I had to experience that too, because - well, there are many reasons, but one reason, is that I had to learn that there are people like Hans, because I would otherwise trust too much... But it was so important to experience that because we all have to go through different stages in the human experience.

There are no "good" or "bad" souls; actually, it's all just an experience. It's like saying "good person - bad thing." You have to have all these different experiences because those are later contained as a memory in your soul. And then, when you are placed into your new identity and into your task, and into a higher evolved state, then you start to realize subconsciously you have all these memories stored, like I had stored as Mousy. (The fear of water was stored) in a big way, a huge storage, but we also have tiny storages that accompany us through life, which kind of buzz and huzz over and around us.

All these different cell memories we carry with us - from all these cellular memories, in Earthly incarnations and others, they help us to be more compassionate and to sense and feel and open our hearts. Because otherwise we wouldn't have those resources we need and we would judge.

NOTE: This reference to cellular memories is repeated in other sessions. Apparently, the memories in question are bits of energy that are stored with us from lifetime to lifetime. Later, there's a description of these stored memories as geometrical shapes that are examined and cleaned between lives. These memories are described as being the "ball bearings" that help us get through our various lifetimes, because we always have access to them – not consciously of course, but through some energetic mechanism that keeps us abreast of them.

LEARNING TO ELIMINATE TIES TO HER FEAR OF WATER

So we carry these memories back so we can learn from them?

No, we bring these memories back because we have them stored. It's so amazing, I've never seen that before, it's like they're stored in your energy field - even in your physical body you have all that in tiny little increments, in little parts... You have that energy stored, and this is why you have access to these huge facets of emotions and feelings, or else we would only be one or two dimensional.

I understand. Are you ready to release the fear of drowning that you have in this lifetime? I would like you to stand with your guide and move into the threads of all those lifetimes where drowning has been an issue with you... How many threads do you see?

Eight.

I want you to take a deep breath and break these threads, and break the fear - it doesn't mean you'll lose the memories, but you can release the emotion, the imprint from those fears of drowning. Move forward and break them.
That (lifetime) was the heaviest one.

Feel the release from your body.
They're gone. (Sighs)

Feel the clearing and cleansing and repairing and restoring that part of you permanently. Let me know when that's complete.
He shows me this big clock; he's always making fun. He showed me this huge alarm clock, with this huge movement; that was his message for me to be patient, the body needs time to understand.

Time to return to this lifetime... Back to where we find ourselves now. Moving back into this room. When you wake on the count of ten, you'll remember all that's happened."
The conversation continued after her session.

RM: That was interesting, the mentioning of the energy around you.
SK: Yes, now I know I'm not hallucinating when I see it. After I've done LBL work in a facilitated state, sometimes I saw these tiny little sparkled dots in colors, and now I know this is the storage from the different incarnations,[16] from the spirit realm, from wherever we were in different incarnations. And now I start to understand why we would carry such an imprint over to that extent. (My drowning in a previous life) was a huge imprint, and I found out that I was this "Negative person" in Hans' life - a bad person, just being concerned about my own well-being, not caring if someone else would die. It's only here on Earth we judge that as something negative - you have to have that experience in order to be compassionate here, in order to really understand why some people are in that experience and then in order to understand there is no such thing as a bad soul. Like you say in therapy, you don't say you are a bad person, it's good person, bad thing what you did.

So I really understood that, linking these lives together and seeing how someone would take on the sacrifice, when the contract is a sacrifice. Shaking the hand of the man who kills you - that was how I was shown that was really a contract to see that he would let me drown so that I would get that lesson and then I was carried over to now a hundred years later. This lifetime. I understand that I had to make the link.

---

[16] In ensuing chapters "energy packets" are reported in a number of life between live sessions.

The following day, Sophia told me that night she had a dream about swimming. She said that prior to her session, a dream of swimming would have been a nightmare, but in this dream she was with her spirit guide, and the two of them were swimming for hours. A few months later, I accompanied her and her then fiancé, now husband Paul Aurand to the beach in Westport, Connecticut. She told me that she felt she had recovered from her fear of water, "nearly 100%."

Is it possible we can cure illnesses by using hypnotherapy to address them? Paul Aurand said his patient was cured after remembering drowning. Michael Newton's patient's shoulder was cured when he remembered being killed in World War I. Later, therapist Debra Haynie recounts a child whose anger issues disappear after remembering being tarred and feathered. Sophia Kramer cures herself of her fear of water after seeing multiple lifetimes where it affected her. These are just a handful of examples.

This form of hypnotherapy could revolutionize medicine, if it's ever studied fully. One can argue that the results negate whether or not the patient is actually remembering a past life or not. As Paul Aurand said: "Who cares?" If you have an unnatural fear of objects, or events, wouldn't you want to find a way to examine it fully? And what of other illnesses? Is it possible to use a journey to the super conscious to heal a patient? As we've seen, numerous patients with psychosomatic illnesses are cured by doing past life regressions. In Chapter 12, a client remembers his father stabbing him in his back, and his lifelong kidney problem disappears. Would it be possible to cure someone of cancer in the future by delving into a past life?

Apparently those that are called to this work are sometimes contacted by patients who have a specific message to them from the spirit world.

"Of course you don't die. Nobody dies. Death doesn't exist. You only reach a new level of vision, a new realm of consciousness, a new unknown world."

- Henry Miller

Chapter 6
TAKE ME TO THE BOOK I NEED TO READ

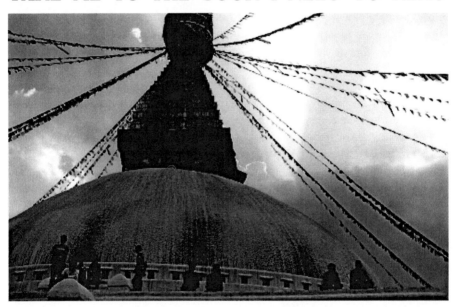

Death ... is no more than passing from one room into another. But there's a difference for me, you know. Because in that other room I shall be able to see.

- Helen Keller

I interviewed Peter Smith to see what he thought of his session with Sophia, and how he came upon the work. Peter is a hypnotherapist who grew up in Melbourne, Australia. Sandy haired with blue eyes, he runs the Newton organization in Australia. I caught Peter just after he'd gone through his own LBL session.

RM: Reflecting on your own LBL - what was your experience today?
PS: I did some more work with the new students, and sometimes we have them work with us, and I was taken back to a past life experience. It was an American Indian life, in fact, and I was in the village when it was invaded by "the white men" and I saw my wife killed. It was quite an interesting experience for me to have those emotions trapped in the soul come forward. You get a bit of a rush with that.

I've got a very strong image of horses bearing down on her and her being killed and how that loss forced me to walk forward and say "Take me also." Which they did. I have a strong image of three bullets plunging into my chest and that was it for me. It was time for me to head home, as many of us did that day.

What do you think you learned in that lifetime?
I went and spoke to my guide, and chatted about that lifetime - it was really about balance, being the very strong masculine Indian hunter which was my specialty, balanced with my spiritual side and also how we were living in harmony with the planet. So the balance of those three is probably a good model for existence at any time, particularly given the way the planet's headed with pollution, global warming and the damage we've done.

What else do you remember about that lifetime?
Animal skins, small pieces of leather holding the hair back; I was not a well-dressed Native American. One thing that stuck out were the warm furs wrapped around my lower legs, which leads me to believe it was in one of the colder climates - I'm not up on native American history, but wonder if that's something I can check into.[17]

TAKE ME TO THE BOOK I NEED TO READ

What about you? Where did you grow up, and did you have any experience with ESP?
I was born and bred in Sydney. Growing up, I had a terrific childhood from a loving and supportive family, and one experience I remember is a really strong dream when I was a young teenager of drifting up and out of my body and looking down at the house. It put me on a path of looking into UFO's and Bigfoot, and all that other stuff. When I got into my 30's, I came across books on past life regression and reincarnation; you read those and think there might be something else here.

---

[17] Many American tribes wore fur leggings, Algonquin, and the Sinkiuse who fought in the Yakima Indian War of 1855. The "Battle of Four Lakes" was fought in September 1858, where 500 Native Americans were hunted down and killed.

I went to live in Melbourne, found a past life regressionist and thought "I'll have a look at this." I went in to get some understanding of what my life really meant. I'd worked in business for many years, ultimately it led me to want to become a hypnotherapist, to try and help other people take that exploration.

After I graduated as a hypnotherapist, I walked into a book store to buy a book for a friend, a professor at a local college. I stood in front of the book shelf, closed my eyes and said "take me to the book I need today." I stepped forward and pulled "Journey of Souls" off the shelf. I guess I forgot to say "take me to the right book for *him*." (Laughs) When you finally come across the reason for what you're here to do, you find it just inspires you to take the next step.

The confirmation I should pursue this work came from the hypnotherapist friend who I bought the book for. He called and said "I have this really strange client. I was doing some work with her, and she went off to this place – it was a room full of knowledge with these beautiful big gold pillars and it sounds like that book you loaned me, but which I never fully read... Can you take her on?" So I said, "Sure."

She came into my clinic, and we went back to the gold pillars using the process we use in hypnotherapy to free-associate with the previous session, and she told me all about the journey of her soul. There was validation of all the things I'd learned; the soul group, the life purpose, she talked to me about a particular karmic pattern across five lifetimes that she had with her current husband.

They were getting a divorce and had beautiful children - she couldn't understand the level of pain she was having. We went into the spiritual realm and her voice and mannerisms changed, and she was able to give me understanding how across five lifetimes she and her husband had these continuing problems. It's then you ask them what they need to do to break that pattern; she said all she needed to do was to forgive him. Afterwards, she had this understanding from her session, and she was able to do that. She had been on her way into a custody battle and everything changed from the fact that she could look him in the eye and finally forgive him after five lifetimes. And her life blossomed after that, she was radiant, a new person. She'd let go of something she'd held onto through lifetimes that no longer held her back. A great outcome.

Were there any doubts you had about the work?
I'd read many things and hadn't agreed with all of them, so I really needed to validate for myself this was happening. I asked her if she'd ever read any books on the topic, she said "No," and then I asked if she'd ever heard of Michael Newton and she said "No." I asked "Well, have you ever had any experience like this before?" She said "No, not since that other therapist and I stumbled upon it a few weeks ago." For me that was authenticity - it must be real. I traveled to America and was trained by the Newton Institute.

A TYPICAL LBL SESSION

Who typically contacts you for an LBL session?
People are drawn from a common desire of wanting to know what's deep within. These sessions normally come about in a person's life where they're ready to explore more about what is within them. Many are on a journey to discover who they are and these sessions answer questions about "Why am I here?" It can happen to anybody at any stage in their life; from corporate executives who run their own businesses, musicians, and people in the alternative health industry, academics; all of these people are drawn to the work for their own reasons. It's a great common denominator.

Any experiences you can recall or share?
To learn that you've been with someone many, many times can be very reassuring, because it gives the knowledge death is really a myth and that they will meet again.

What do you think they take away from an LBL?
A number of things; my life's purpose, the lineage of my soul. Fear of death evaporates and you gain an understanding of those you may have lost in this life are not far away, and that there's great shared experiences over many lifetimes. It puts you in touch with a realm of absolute peace and love and compassion. To realize that is waiting for all of us when it's time for us to head home - that is the most reassuring news I think anyone can ever have.

I think traditional belief systems are breaking down all over the world; people are looking for something more, for a greater understanding of themselves, rather than being told by other people what to believe. If you can look at what you have within, that's got to be the real stuff because it's your own. If you can tap into that, have access to that, it's very empowering. The world is picking up pace and if we can have something that's centering, like an awakening and understanding of your immortal identity, that seems to be the most centering you could ever have. The more people discover the beautiful compassion and wisdom we hold within, that's got to be good for the planet.

I met with the man in charge of vetting of the applicants for the Michael Newton Institute's accreditation through their conferences. Jimmy E. Quast[18] holds a doctorate degree in Clinical Hypnotherapy from the American Institute of Hypnotherapy .[19] He does a rigorous amount of quality control to ensure that those who apply are serious hypnotherapists with a successful track record of helping patients. A man with an easy smile and a dry sense of humor, his southern roots pepper the tone of his calm voice and demeanor.

---

[18] www.eastonhypnosis.com.
[19] Accredited by California's State Department of Education

RM: How did you come upon this work and this field of Michael's work?
Dr. Jimmy Quast: It was not my profession originally, my degree is in education, and I was forty years old when I went back to school and became a hypnotherapist. When Dr. Newton needed some people to learn how to do his work so he could retire, I was one of the people asked to help him teach that first group.

I was very skeptical at first. I didn't buy the premise of between lives therapy. It wasn't that I didn't believe in spiritual things, I was doing past life work, I just didn't trust Dr. Newton's approach. But a woman asked if I would do one of these 'between life' sessions, and I agreed, because she hadn't read any of his books, she knew nothing about it. I figured she wouldn't know any of it and that would be my proof so I could wash my hands of the whole thing!

But when she went into a trance, she knew everything Dr. Newton wrote about, the soul group, the council. She sat up in my therapy chair in a deep, super conscious state and said "Jimmy, listen up there's some things you need to know." She explained things to me very lovingly, took me under her wing and just told me the truth. She could pull up any topic I wanted and give me more details. You could say my jaw was between the heels of my shoes and the electric current I felt in my spine was near a point where you could be electrocuted. I was in shock.

She spoke of the soul group and how that's constructed, the council of elders, and how they function and what their nature is, and we met her spirit guide. Because of all the details she knew, I knew I had been wrong. I had misjudged Dr. Newton too. She had come for my benefit; this wasn't a session for her. There's nowhere to go after something like that happens to you. It changes you forever.

What kind of stuff did she say to you?
She verified it in detail, exactly the way Dr. Newton wrote about it, having never read his material. After that session, she disappeared, I never saw her again. We have names for that kind of soul, one that comes out of nowhere because you need something. They touch your life and they're on their way. She knocked me

out of my limited belief system, my disbelief, you could say, of all that Dr. Newton spent much of his life accumulating. I knew then he really was a scientist, he had been carefully collecting this data for years, 7000 cases and it was to be taken to heart. I started pulling clients' names out of my file whom I thought might benefit from this sort of work. They had marvelous experiences too, and I was off and running. There was no turning back.

A TYPICAL LBL SESSION

What's a typical session?
It usually starts on the telephone or by email and I will ask what the person's intentions are, if there's some issues, they're going to be with me a minimum of three hours, and sometimes a lot more - four or five or even six hours. Once we achieve the right depth and the client starts speaking, if we're lucky they're a soul that has been incarnating for quite a while and they know what they're up to and we just scramble to keep up with them. But more often than not, they need help, a lot of encouragement and it will be like pulling teeth - you need a lot of patience.

"YOU'VE GOT TO GO BACK"

Anything surprise you?
The most surprising one was a very short session. This person had a job which made her very uncomfortable, because she was in a leadership position, head of a corporation and it was very stressful for her. Turned out she was a very experienced soul; she had already finished incarnating in her last life. We began her session with the death scene from her previous life, and as she's moving away from the Earth, having all the normal sensations and things she's reporting, all of a sudden she's met by a group of friends saying "You've got to go back." This didn't mean to go back to the body that just died; apparently there was no way to do that. I didn't know what was going on, but you just stay with it.

Pretty soon she's at the gateway and sees her guide and he's saying "Come on!" and she's saying to him, "No, I have to go back." And these two friends, who had met her, were preparing her to get into a stream of energy, they had found a fetus that would have been a still born baby - I don't want to upset anybody's belief system, but this is what we're told consistently by thousands of souls - it was one of those babies. So this baby was going to be an unoccupied vehicle unless she returned.

Usually there's a great deal of planning that goes on before a lifetime, with all of your friends and loved ones who are going to be involved with you. You have to seriously think about the type of body and brain that are most compatible with you, or that might challenge you - these are all parameters we consider, and also how much of our soul energy you're going to put in. You never put all of it in, as part of our energy is always at home in the spirit world, which is true for all of us. A human body couldn't sustain all of our energy. I know that I have 20% for example, because I've had my own LBL, which means I'm running a little low on fuel and I know it.

But this woman took that stream of energy and sped right back into a fetus and made it fit. This was a real task and if she hadn't been a very experienced soul I doubt it would have been done, and the result wasn't really a wonderful fit. So here she was a grown woman as I meet her and she's suicidal. Very intelligent, she's got a number of degrees, but she's one very intelligent and unhappy person.

She was finished incarnating you understand, she didn't have to come back, she only came back because she'd made a promise to someone she loved. It was so touching, this session was already over and I was there saying "Wait, we haven't gotten there yet." But she understood what had happened and said "I get it now. It all makes sense. I can do this now. I'm okay."

NO ONE HORDES THE BEANS

And the structure of the spirit world remains uniform?
It's not just a few clouds and people playing harps, it's a very complex, you could say society, and one in which there are none of the human limitations. We don't have the human needs, nobody can horde the jelly beans, and there is no power to horde. There's not really a hierarchy, although you have advanced souls and beginner souls, but souls don't see that as a hierarchy. Part of becoming an advanced soul is to become more selfless and humble; they don't see themselves as more important or special than the youngest of souls. All souls look up to others.

It's really about self-advancement and helping everyone else advance, unlike the physical world where you can advance by stepping on people - you can't do that there. You advance by doing something positive, testing yourself and overcoming your limitations, or by helping somebody else to advance. Help them, help you.

Quantum physics explains that everything physical and solid is, in fact, just pure energy. So you're shifting to an existence in which objects or structures are of a higher order of energy than on Earth. And there is infinite space and the only lack is the desire to perfect ourselves. We seem to want to reach a level of self-perfection that will allow us to somehow get back to the source that gave us our existence in the first place. If you want to use a religious term, "we're trying to get back to God" as souls.

Just as humans can't tell you what God is, the most experienced souls we can talk to - ones that are still incarnating - they'll laugh if you ask "Could you explain God to me?" They call that "the presence," or "the source." They know what you mean when you say God, of course, and they'll tell you, "I can't tell you what that is;" but they say they can feel it.

As souls, we feel that presence. It's around us, we're enveloped by it, especially in special places in the spirit world, like with the Elders; it's very strong there. But we can't explain what it is even at that level, so how are we going to do so as human beings, trying to describe God?"

"There are things you need to know." Jimmy was skeptical, didn't really buy the whole premise of 'between lives' therapy. But then, a client appeared out of the blue who made a believer out of Jimmy. Currently he's the person who checks the therapy credentials of those who attend Newton Institute conferences and are seeking becoming certified members of the Michael Newton Institute.

But as you'll see, if Jimmy hadn't found the patient that led him to Newton or hadn't been so damned good at what he does; I wouldn't be writing this sentence.

I believe we are reincarnated. You, I, we reincarnate over and over. We live many lives, and store up much experience. Some are older souls than others and so they know more. It seems to be an intuitive "gift." It is really hard-won experience.

- Henry Ford

Chapter 7
VANUM POPULATUM

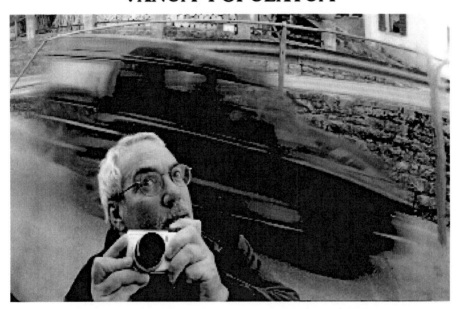

"Vanum; Emptiness, hollow, Vanity. Populatum: To Lay Waste, Ravage. To utterly destroy, to annihilate, to wipe from the face of the Earth."

- Definition of a Latin phrase overheard during a dream.

I was waking up in our penthouse in Santa Monica when I heard someone whisper in my ear "Vanum Populatum." I wrote it down on a piece of paper and left it there to explore later. Some days later, I ran across it, and started to wonder *Who was trying to speak to me in Latin?* I don't know Latin, never studied it, however I did toy with being an altar boy in our local Catholic Church. (Alas, a week after I'd memorized the Latin Mass, they switched to English.)

But I had the curious impression it was *me* talking to me in this dead language, albeit an older version of me. I found an online dictionary and discovered vanum is actually a word in Latin. It means "vanity." Populatum means "To annihilate completely, to utterly destroy, to wipe off the face of the Earth." I was startled. "Who wants me to annihilate vanity?" After all I live in L.A., Vanity Central. Where do I start?

But also I realized the phrase carried essentially the same meaning as the Buddhist concept "Destroy the Ego." Yet it carried a different meaning than the traditional "annihilation of the delusion of self under philosophical examination" in Buddhist philosophy. "Destroy Egotism" is to destroy things of the self which are hollow, or have no meaning – the trappings of vanity. Accolades, notoriety or fame, or even success as it's known in societal terms; the big house, the fast car, the media attention; not just to deny those things – but to annihilate them.

When I was offered the opportunity to have my own past life/life between life sessions, I knew I should bring a list of questions. They could be anything, and if one went deep enough, they could be the answer to any question one might have about the afterlife. However, since I'd never been hypnotized, I was wary the therapist might lead me – so I added a trick question. "What is the meaning of vanum populatum?" I'm probably the only person on the planet who would know the answer to that question and nearly impossible for a hypnotist to lead me to it.

After filming a number of sessions, Paul Aurand suggested I film my own session. I was a fan of George Plimpton's work, injecting himself into the various themes he wrote about, and despite wanting to remain objective, I knew there was only one way for me to see what the people I was filming were experiencing.

However, I had little confidence I could be hypnotized. I'm fairly aware of whenever there's a camera in the room, and being a filmmaker, spend a fair amount of brain power thinking about what it's seeing. The worst that could happen would be having hours of footage of me saying "I'm sorry, it's not working."

The following is a transcript of my session with Jimmy Quast, who, as mentioned, has an easy smile with a sparkle in his eyes, a soft southern accent and a swath of grey in his auburn hair.

Being hypnotized is unlike "stage hypnosis" where a performer snaps his or her fingers and gets the subject to participate in a group trance. This felt more like a 'guided meditation,' something I've done before in India and Tibet with the help of Robert Thurman. I was fully conscious throughout, awake and aware – even used the facilities a couple of times over the four hours we spent together. And I was also conscious of the camera filming me on a couch, as Jimmy sat in a chair next to me, a notebook in his lap.

After a half hour or so of talking me into a calm state, *("You're floating in the water near a Caribbean island with warm water…")* Jimmy began to take me back in time.

Jimmy Quast: "You're in your front yard, 12 years old. What color is this house?"
Me: I'm in the front yard making a bow and arrow. (I saw my home as it looked in 1967, older cars in the driveways of homes nearby) I've got an ax – Oh. I've cut my finger deeply. (I saw blood coming out of my finger) I've cut through the skin, it's deep, bleeding and I have to get my dad. (I choked up at the sight of my father, who had passed away a few years earlier. I was also profoundly aware of my 12 year old emotion of seeing him, the rescuer who can solve any problem.)

He's washing it now - we're inside at the sink. And then we go to the doctor to stitch it up… he's telling me never to point the ax toward me… "Always away." Something I remember through life.

When he's there with you, helping you, how does that feel?
He really knows how to take care of things. He's a smart guy.

What's the house like?
The house is a single floor; at this point I'm sharing a room with my brother Robbie… (As I spoke, I saw Robbie, a red headed, freckle faced brother about 17.)

What's in your room?
Bunk beds. Stickers on the closet door from Mad magazine. There's writing on the bunk bed underneath… (I was looking at the bottom panel of the top bunk) I can see my brothers and I have written graffiti on the bottom of the bed.

Anything special in this room?
A Tibetan Thankga my uncle gave to my dad. He found it in Burma during World War II, I didn't realize until I was an adult what it was.

Any place else?
My mom's a concert pianist, so there's a piano in the living room, set against a beautiful red brick wall. Downstairs is a basement with all of my father's tools - it's where my father works as an architect and it smells like lead pencils.

Let's go deeper and younger…
It's the hospital… I'm… coming out… (I gasp). I'm being born. I see the doctor's face with this thing on his head - it's bright and he's sort of - not whacking me - I guess I'm breathing okay - his face is the first thing I see. I can see him clearly,

the color of his eyes, the mask on his head, the head banded metal thing that's reflecting light, the mask across his mouth - intense hazel eyes. It's very clear. It's a little bit cold... now he's placed me with her and it's nice to be with my mom. It's startling to see... such bright lights.

Let's go back a step; to before you were born... you're in your mother's womb now, into the womb, any impressions coming to you?
I hear voices, but like a buzz. I hear her heartbeat... pleasant. My body is working ok, fairly comfortable here, my mom is happy... I'm just in tune with her.

Anything else you pick up on?
My dad's not at my birth. He's driving here. I'm aware of the logistics of he's not here, she is; he's on his way. [20]

Go back... getting younger and smaller, traveling with speed perhaps... Back and back, guided to another time, a different place. A different life; one that would be most beneficial to you, the one just before this life of Rich. I want you to trust the impressions without editing or analyzing. What are the impressions?
NOTE: I paused for some time, seeing and saying nothing. I didn't want to "satisfy the questioner" that I remembered a past life if I really didn't. I was fully prepared to say "I don't see anything," and end the session. I felt obligated to be skeptical of "seeing" something that I didn't actually see. So time passed, while I scanned in my mind's eye, for any kind of visual. Nothing came to me, until Jimmy said simply "Just look down."

MY PAST LIFE AS AN AMERICAN INDIAN

Just look down. What do you see?
This is unusual. (I saw my bare feet in a creek. The water was cold, soothing. My feet bloody, scratched.) What's coming to me is... Native American Indian. I'm a male. And I'm trying to get the impression here... What's on my legs? I want to say buckskin, there's a feather. Two feathers, not up, but down... tied in my hair, black hair, and I can feel my clothing - suede vest, pants... bare feet. [21]

How old are you?
Seems like 28. I'm looking around; it's hills, trees and dried old grass. It's the dry season...

---

[20] After this session, I spoke to my mother and asked her where dad was while I was being born, and she said, "He was driving on his way to the hospital..." something I had not known previously.

[21] I found out later from a Lakota historian that medicine men had two feathers pointing down.

Are you alone?
Not around anyone else at the moment – I'm by a creek; I can put my foot in. I have wounds on my feet; don't know why, but... I notice they're beaten up, feels good to put them in the water.

Is that why you've come here?
I come here for solace to get away. I think it's about my spirit guide. I come here to commune.

A spiritual connection with your guide... what do they call you?
I heard Tan' tanka' mon, I think that means "running bear" which sounds funny to me; tatanka... (Remembering the Kevin Costner film "Dances With Wolves," where he was a Lakota Sioux named "Buffalo" – Tatanka). In my case it means "Runs from bear." It might be Watanka...[22]

Your spirit guide is here by the water?
Not a human guide. It's a cougar.[23] Mountain lion.

What does that mean to you?
Hunter, alone.

Would it be okay to visit where your people are?
(Sigh) I'd prefer not to.

Where is your village?
My overall impression is that... it's gone. (Sigh)

Just relax... (Puts his hand on my forehead)
I see. I didn't want to tell you about it. There's a wife, involved... there was a problem.

You're safe, tell me what happened.
(I started to choke up. In my mind's eye a village of teepees and bodies everywhere. A massacre. Lots of blood. People hacked to death.)

What happened?
Hacked to death.

---

[22] Tatanka, means "Bull Buffalo" in Lakota. According to my historian, it's definitely a Lakota name. Watanka means "Great Spirit."
[23] Some Native American tribes have a "Vision Quest" where they commune with an animal spirit, who becomes their "spirit guide."

By whom?
Damned Hurons. [24] Everyone's dead.

Except you?
(Through tears) I was away. I was doing something else, picking something up. I just came back and everyone is dead.

Your wife?
Yes.

NOTE: In my mind's eye, I saw this village of massacred Indians whom I sincerely believed to be my people. I went to a teepee, the classical type with a leather flap and sticks holding it up, and pulled it aside to see a beautiful woman with long black hair lying in a pool of blood, dead. I was overwhelmed with the emotion of seeing her; my dead wife. But I was also conscious of the fact that this emotion swept over me – If I was making this up, why was I so connected to this emotion? I started to sob.

I had one child... My son was taken. (Feeling the full emotion of that thought.)

And where do you go now? Do you have any place?
That's why I'm here, by the river, soaking my feet. I'm trying to understand.

I want you to move to your last day in this life. In this body. Are you still alone?
I'm alone. I see. It's alcohol and drowning. I got drunk and went to the river and just slipped away. (A muddy brown river, floating down, holding a whisky bottle, bobbing like a cork.)

Not much else to do, was there?
No. Everything about my life that I cared for - my family, my culture, my world is gone.

Move away from that body. You're free now. Are you looking back?
Much happiness.

You feel any remorse?
No, I'm just passing into "the Great White." I've done this many times. It's time to move home. No reason to linger.

NOTE: Some years ago, I was at a Christmas party with some old friends, and they pulled out a bottle of whisky from 1840 that had been in the family for generations. We all took a sip of this concoction, which was smooth and burning at the same time – nothing like modern day liquor. At that moment I had a flash of me holding an old empty whisky bottle.

---

[24] My conscious mind thought - "If I'm calling myself by a Sioux name, I couldn't be fighting with a tribe associated with the East Coast." But post session, I discovered through research that the Sioux and the Huron fought a series of battles in the upper Midwest.

A JOURNEY TO THE LIFE BETWEEN LIVES

Tell me what this is like, you're moving away.
Going home? Looking ahead. Just getting together with my friends. (I saw a vast field of white in the distance, then I moved into it at lightning speed until the faces and bodies came into full focus. A crowd of people greet me). They're here with me... It's just lovely. Lots of friends. Smiling. Embracing me. Everybody's here.

Recognize anyone?
My wife. (The Indian one; long black hair, and a young boy next to her. A profound sense of connection with them.)

The one who was killed.
My son. Both of them. (I saw them standing together, smiling at me).

Who else?
My father. (Charles, who passed away in 2004.)

How are they arranged?
Sort of a semi-circle. About 20 or so.

Who comes out of this group first?
An elder. Comes out from the center, about twelve o'clock. A male, white hair, somebody very gentle, welcoming me, he's my grandfather at one point... (Not in this life - He has a kindly, old face, very distinct, about 70 years old. Smiling. A warm greeting)

His immortal name?
Ray... ma.

Does he touch you? How does that feel like?
Fabulous.

Does Rayma have any message for you?
"Welcome home. Welcome... *home*." Nice.

Back to the circle, welcoming you. Any colors?
Purple light. That's his light.

If you were to rate this in terms of brightness... is it bright?
Deep purple, rich purple.

Is Rayma your personal teacher?
Feels like it; he seems to be in charge.

So the others, is there a different color?
It seems like everyone's sort of in a darker blue.

NOTE: In Michael Newton's "Destiny of Souls" he catalogs soul colors of the Afterlife by asking "If I held up a mirror, what color would you be?" He learned the categories followed those from a prism of light; youngest, white, moving to darker colors, the eldest, purple.

MY SOUL GROUP

What's your sense of this group? Is this your own family? Or is this different?
I sense I'm hanging out with them all the time. It's a little odd that I'm not seeing people come forward, just one, but I sense they're my group. (Seeing a semi-circle of light. When one light moved forward, his features came into view)

If you could see you, through their vision, what do you look like?
Dark blue. Purple's on the outside, blue is sort of interspersed, like strings, like stripes, they sort of move back and forth. It's not a static color, it sort of moves. Rayma seems to be a dark purple.

Is there someplace he'd like to take you?
He wants to take me to a healing center.

How does he do that?
Just sort of glides me by the hand, I know where to go, we go together. It's like an energy field, if you looked at it, you'd see it as multiple, colored lights, but depending what work needs to be done, it's just you and your light. It's sort of the way I was sitting by the river, same kind of equipoise where you draw energy from the room into places where it's been depleted.

NOTE: A common occurrence in sessions, where a person goes to a "place of healing." In my mind's eye, this center was a room filled with energy. I walked into this room and sat down so I could go through the "re-energizing process." It's difficult to describe with words, other than perhaps being re-energized in a Star Trek transporter. As I used my mind to draw energy into me, it was as if I was filling myself with liquid, and all the areas that had been depleted from a difficult life as an American Indian, now were being made whole again.

Anyone assisting you?
Just him, he's observing as I pull the energy into myself. Mentally you draw the energy towards you to repair the places that are damaged or missing. It feels like filling up with liquid water, but blissful water, filling you as you pull it to the places that need to be healed. I'm aware there are people that can do that for you, but you can do it yourself.

You don't need those people to help you?
I don't think so, because Rayma's just sort of smiling and enjoying it.

How long does this process carry on?
The idea is to go from the floor up, (Pictured myself sitting, with feet on the ground, energy coming in waves through my feet to my head) you move it from your toes to your head and then back down repeatedly because each time more energy comes forward. It's a process, doesn't seem to take long. Afterwards you feel rejuvenated.

Is Rayma involved where you're going next?
I'm asking him where we are going next and he said "Well, that's up to you." A bit of comedy.

Where do you want to go next?
I want to go see my friends.

What does Rayma say to that?
"Let's go!" Oh, there's so many places you can go here, people you can see, they're everywhere...

Strewn about?
Well it's more organized, but there are many opportunities to stop and see people and friends and those you've touched before.

Do you have a core group that you started out with at one time?
I do. For some reason I feel like they're out working and doing their own thing. My core group is teachers and I can go visit them in their classes.
    NOTE: In my mind's eye, this classroom was like anyone I've been in, or taught in; students in rows at their desks, sitting down, the teacher standing in front of them, some kind of blackboard, or smart board behind them. In this case, I recognized one of the teachers as an old friend of mine – I knew her name, but didn't recognize her as anyone that I've met in this lifetime. She had blond hair, and a bright, white essence about her.

A TRIP TO AN ENERGY CONSTRUCTION CLASSROOM

What's going on?
Just greetings and salutations. I'm in a classroom with a friend who's a teacher and she's introducing me. The teacher knows me but the class doesn't.

You're like a guest speaker?
Her name is Kajeera, she teaches a class in... Energy construction.

Do you know about that?

She says I do. Energy construction has to do with aligning energy, aligning the milk of the universe into geometric shapes. They retain energy, they retain everything, the stuff of the universe; memories, dreams, reflections, attitudes, happiness, joy; composed of physical stuff mostly - containing emotions, because emotion is energy, so when you have an intention, it goes into this geometric shape and it stays there.. And if you create it properly it will stay there.

NOTE: These shapes are similar to the ones Sophia mentions in her session recounted in "Aquaphobia," and similar to the packets of energy mentioned in Morrin's session in "Golden Light Within."

You can keep the energy in the geometric shape?

Right, but also you're retaining it. So let's say you're in the classroom and you create this energy; you put your good intention (or some kind of intention) together into this geometric shape. You bring it to life, and you create it so that it stays with you and then you're able to carry that energy packet into your current life so you can have access to it.

That's why it's important to bring it along with you -- how else are you going to retain all of your past experiences unless you have these energy fields? (Responding to Kajeera holding up an example) I see. Here's the thing, you're in the classroom...--I'm starting to sound like a teacher --

Maybe you are...

You're in the classroom and your teacher helps you to manipulate energy, that's the basic thing - the actual things you're creating in the classroom are almost like emotional ball bearings...

That's the geometrical part?

Yes, they do have different shapes. But because the nature of the way it's designed, it looks like a geometric shape - but that's how it functions. Try to think of it as a ball bearing - we know how ball bearings work, they help everything in a machine move more fluidly - so you carry these ball bearings with you through your incarnations. And as you go along, unfortunately, they pick up negative energy, and that causes disruption in the ball bearings. So when you come back here, you work on cleaning that stuff up - make new ball bearings, restructure them - like taking them into the shop.

So Kajeera teaches people how to do that?

She does.

What's the level of this class? New souls?

No, I can tell you their colors are white tinged with gold. They've been around a bit, but they're learning how to manipulate energy for retention later, it's a lovely class. (pause) I'm praising her, how lucky they are to have such a great teacher.

Is that why Rayma brought you here?
He said it was up to me, I was in charge of that. I get a feeling he's treating me like I'm somehow... he's sort of like a friend traveler, more than like a spirit guide.... it's unusual.

Even though he's this take charge guy.
Well I mean he's the most vocal. Because he's got the most energy in that area, he feels comfortable speaking up, but I sense he's treating me in a very gracious way, that I'm part of his group or something - it's just very honored and flattered by it.

NOTE: I've never talked or thought about geometric shapes retaining "life energy" or "Memories of a lifetime" but it mirrors what quantum physicists have posited about consciousness possibly existed outside the body. I've seen a ball bearing, but not since I was a kid sneaking into the local car shop to look at the pin-up calendars and pretending I needed one.

A TRIP TO A HEALING CENTER CLASS

And you're just visiting friends like Kajeera... Where are we heading next?
He's asking me "Where do you want to go?" I'm telling him I'd like to go see Luana's class. (As I entered the "classroom" I saw her as a young blond in her 20's, years before I met her – wearing a pony tail, with bright blond hair sitting in the back of the class.) She's in a healing class.

Oh, this is a *deep* class. She's part of a group of older souls and her teacher is incredibly smart. Their job is to help people on the planet... Earth. And when they do energy work on Earth... wow. So they're able to help people.

How do they do that?
They heal humans. I'm asking them "How are the candidates chosen?" (I had the sense of being in a classroom where everyone in the class turns to look at you, wondering what you're doing there). Not sure they want to tell me. Wait, let me just ask. (Pause) Well it's the choosing. How are they chosen? (In my mind's eye, the class wasn't used to being interrupted, and the teacher is patient, but not particularly pleased I've interrupted them. I saw Luana smiling in the back, looking mildly amused by the discomfort.)

Are they holding back because I'm here?
No, they're saying the choosing of the candidates is a very complex process, but Luana's trying to explain that the easy way to say it would be if somebody was really in need of spiritual help and they focused their mind on asking for help... (Pause) It's like they (members of the class) would help a healer, somebody here on the planet that is a healing energy person who calls upon them to help, and they come

down, or come here and supply the energy, the light, to help the healing process.[25]

However, there are caveats - it gets complicated because some people aren't supposed to have the help when they ask for it, because it hinders their journey, so that's where it becomes a little complex.

They have to be ready and ask...
That's right. But this is a very playful, fun class, everybody here is very talented and highly evolved and I'm really only allowed in because I'm seeing Luana, my friend, who I knew in this life.

And Rayma?
He's not present. I'm trying to focus on the teacher.

What's your connection to Luana? Is she one of your old bunch?
I'm getting the sense we've had many lifetimes together - but way back - a long time ago. We came together this lifetime after many interruptions. I'm getting the sense I've done that with many people.

NOTE: In the last chapter, I revisit this detail, and through the help of my spirit guide, detail a life where I claim she and I were part of a Sumerian cult. I hasten to add I know little about Sumeria, have less information about Sumerian Priests or cults, but I reference it here and examine it later on.

Is Luana a spirit name?
It's close to her spirit name. (Laughs) She's interrupting, she's teasing me. We had so many names with reference to her name Luana; "Zooluaga," "Lufthansa;" people had a hard time with her name, and now she's just having fun with me. She's not going to give it to me.

So aliases are a fun thing...
Well teasing, anyway... But her teacher is a very important person to know. I want to say Teth...era... He's green; he has a deep rich green healing light.

Masculine?
Masculine, no, he's just... that's the sense of him. But he bridges all. Deep green, he's showing me the glowing healing color.

Coming from his center?
It's around him. His center is purple. I wanted to say that I get a sense that even in this life, the people around me haven't been with me in recent lives, but they were in past lives.

---

[25] This process is described later, which I found in various citations about near death experience (NDEs) and LBL's. However, at this point, I'd never heard that Doctors or healers on Earth might have help from the Afterlife.

Looks like judging by their color they may not really be incarnating anymore?
Tethera? No, he's a teacher; he's a full timer (meaning "non reincarnating spirit"). But the students in her class, will be coming back. Luana will be coming back, she may be back already. I'll have to track that.

NOTE: When asked a question I can't answer, I feel myself saying things randomly like "I'll have to track that," as if I had the ability to do so. However, in the later session with another hypnotherapist, I was able to find an answer to that question, and give a detailed answer about Luana's current incarnation on Earth.

WHY I CHOSE THIS LIFETIME

What are you involved with?
My work? It's a form of healing. It involves energy transfer, I'm trying to do it with art, voice, music, film; but I get caught up in so many other things that hold me back from doing that. It's like I'm trying to teach how to transfer energy through emotion, through words, through language, through art.

Everything you create is an energy form, if you create positive energy things, energy forms, then you're putting out positive love and energy into the universe, it's a way of keeping that light going... of expanding it.

So you are in healing as well?
I think it's a form of healing, but this is my odd way of doing it... You can heal people through words. We all know you can heal through action, but the idea of healing through words, through thoughts and putting those into pictures and film, because those are all images of...

Just another way to deliver the energy...
..the same energy, that transfer.

It's very clear to you.
It's clear to me, but (in my career) I'm not very successful at it. What was I thinking?
NOTE: At this point Jimmy laughed, but so did the members of my council. I had the odd experience of getting laughs on two different planes of existence simultaneously.

I mean I've had limited success (in my career), because people are caught up in their own things, their own paths, and there's so much information that's perhaps not healing, that's not in a positive manner, that gets dissipated into the sea of energy transference...

Sounds like you're a little bit frustrated.
I agreed I would come and do this (using healing energy through filmmaking), and that's what I'm doing. It could be I'm just here to help other people have success.

This was Rayma's idea?
My idea. And using Rich (referring to myself as the current vehicle, as if Jimmy was asking the question to my eternal self) to be the story teller.

Have you tried this before in other lives? With the voice, the music?
When I was the Indian, the Native American, I was a healer.

Was that about using herbs...?
No, I was healing through touch. Like a shaman - people accepted I was good at that way of healing - witch doctor, I guess, and they came to me (in the Native American world) when they had psychological problems.

So you're trying something different this time, you're an innovator, looking for another way to...?
Honestly, I don't think it was my original idea, I get the sense that other people are using it right now, on the planet, using voice and energy, and maybe it's always been the case, I think it was just that I was going to try it myself this time. "I'll step up and see if I can do that." Still, I have a certain amount of confidence in my ability to deliver (chuckles) which is unusual.

Did you actually have a teacher who suggested it?
NOTE: As Jimmy asked this question, I saw myself in a "life planning session" - standing in a room full of people, casually sitting around, as I raised my hand and detailed how I was going to attempt a lifetime that dealt with the same kind of energy that's involved in healing, but through cinematic arts. I saw myself describing it as an "outside the box" way of viewing energy transfer between people, and how the healing energy of the Universe can be drawn down in a variety of fashions, including, surprisingly, film, music and art.

It came from a classroom environment, yes, where we were talking about coming back and what was the method you could use to help people with energy transference, that might be a little bit out of the box, or unusual, or different.

Did the word fun come into it?
I think it was just natural I'm fun. I think whatever I ended up doing was going to be fun.

And you've learned that quite well. It seems...
Well, the quickest path from someone's lips to their consciousness is through laughter. Because then they can hear it. Tears work as well, but certainly laughter is the most pleasant way.

Will you continue, are you trying to decide if it's worthwhile..?
I think, I've made the deal -- I'm "in for a penny, in for a pound."

And that's with regard to the life as Rich?
I'm being told it's all going to pan out the way I imagined it. It just takes time. It's one of my bugaboos; patience. I've always charged up the hill expecting everyone to follow and then I turn around and no one's there. And then I go down the hill and say "Hey, what the heck's going on?" they say "Patience. Give us time to get on the same wavelength."

Is this part of your lesson? Patience, is really important?
Yeah, patience is really key... and letting go. There's a lot to be said for enthusiasm, but also a lot to be said for just letting go.

So is it clear to you that patience is going to be essential, from what you're telling me?
Patience, because the end result will work out as I imagined it, and had planned it - and intricately manipulated it. And everyone's on the same ride and I think it's going to work out just fine.

I'm wondering and I'm not sure why... Tatanka...
I said that wrong... either "Tan Tanka" or "Wa' tanka."

   NOTE: Through research, I've been able to determine that Wa'tanka means "Holy Man" in the Lakota language, typically be a name for a Holy or Medicine Man. Tatanka, as we've learned from "Dances with Wolves," means Buffalo. "Tanka" means great, "Tan-tanka" means short. According to R.J. DeMailie, the Dakota world was "characterized by its oneness," with no separation between the natural and supernatural world. Wakan Tanka is defined as "the animating force" of the universe" or "The Great Spirit."

WHY I COMMITTED SUICIDE IN THAT LIFE

He was a healer and his life ended in a way that I wonder if that has imparted some energy... or shift in direction.
(Thinking of the way I saw the death, floating down a big muddy river while drinking a bottle of whisky) A little bit of water filling the lungs is not pleasant; alcohol wasn't really a huge problem, but it certainly a lesson to avoid, but I knew that everything was over, the shell was just there... age.

When you returned from that life as Wa' tanka and the welcome back seems really marvelous, is there any concern about how you brought about your own death?
I would tell you right away if I felt it was a suicide, it really wasn't... it was more just letting... go.

Incredible remorse there, unhappiness because everyone else was gone.
Honestly it was a tired body, and the loss of not only my people, but all the values of my people, and the way a person feels when they've been dominated by another

group to the point of relentlessness. I mean, I sensed it was time to move to the next episode. The journey was finished and it was just time to move on, and I don't think I had the courage to do a sky burial. (Referring to an ancient Lakota practice of leaving the dead on a scaffold for consumption by birds.) Easier to just float down the river.

Easy to get drunk and go in the river.
(Chuckles) Have a little cocktail before you go and then have the big cocktail. And honestly I didn't chastise myself for it. It was just; "Was the ride okay?"

Is there someplace else that we need to go?
NOTE: I continue this thought later in the session, but the research shows there is no pejorative concept associated with a person taking their own life, rather it's the person themselves who is reportedly distraught over breaking previous commitments to complete a chosen life. There's a sacred oath involved with choosing a life, and those who break it return to find themselves disappointed with their lack of ability to fulfill it. In this case, I argue that the life I was leading had become a shell and was ready to return.

A TRIP TO THE COUNCIL OF ELDERS

Let's go to the council.

Does Rayma come along on this trip?
(Pause) He's there with me. He says "You're on." (Like an actor going onstage.)
  NOTE: I had the profound sense of a buzz in the room, as if there was some kind of anticipation of my speaking to the council. The only feeling I can associate it with is just prior to going onstage to perform or speak, but knowing that good friends are in the audience, and eager to participate. In my research, many people had said they were apprehensive about this trip to see their council, either having the feeling like a trip to the principal's office, or in Albert Brook's hilarious "Defending Your Life," before a judge. In my case, it felt fun.

What's this like?
Beautiful room; beautiful in a light sense. A radiant room, radiant place. And... counting (the amount of people in the room)...

The energy, what's that like?
Very peaceful... (Laughs) I feel like it's a little bit of a performance.

By whom?
By me, but because they're used to my sort of antics, everybody's in a good mood. Eight people that I can see. There might be more...

What do they look like?
Non-denominational... sort of just lights.

Not flashy.
No, rich hues of purple and a little bit of red tinge over there. Just purple with a tinge of vermillion... (Seeing a woman cloaked in a purple light, but a few streaks of bright red shining within).

What's the red mean to you?
Fierce... warrior... fierce person. I've got green here, but it's a purple green... [26]What's the color called... chartreuse?

Just checking again, how do you look to them?
That dark blue with maybe a little, I want to say, purple.

It is what it is?
And... I'm asking them my questions.

   NOTE: I'd read that it was helpful for the session to bring a list of questions that might be answered. I had no clue that I would get this far in my own session, but the night before, I quickly jotted down some questions one might ask God if they had the chance. My first questions: "What does Vanum Populatum mean?" was a trick question, as I knew for certain that no one, outside of me, would know the answer. The rest were #2. "What is my connection to Tibet? Or Rome?" – two places I felt that I'd returned to. #3. "What part in my life does music play?" #4. My relationship with Luana. #5. A question about the deaths of my Father and friend Paul Tracey #6 was a question about a vivid dream I had when my daughter Olivia was born, #7 "What creative projects I should focus on?" #8 and finally "What's the meaning of my life, what am I doing here?" Oddly enough, after the session, I thought the therapist had asked the questions and I answered them, but the footage shows that I asked them in my head as if I'd memorized them, even though I'd only jotted them down the night before.
   They're saying... "Yes." (Laughs.) "Yes, you were a monk in Tibet, not so long ago."

Something that you want to pause and go look at it?
It was in a monastery that was an old tradition of Buddhism, closer to the older dogmatic point of view. Nyingma? (One of the older Buddhist sects in Tibet.) They're reminding me this monastery was not as rich in tradition. The reason I was there was to learn patience (laughs) because the teachers were not very bright and I felt I knew more than they did. That particular life, as a Tibetan monk, was to learn patience.[27]

---

[26] Green is associated with being a healing color in many cultures, including Tibetan. (Green Tara)

[27] I examine this more fully in the final chapter.

Is there a pattern with you and patience?
Through eternity. They're also taking me back to my other question. the vanum populatum question; it was a dream that came to me and it was me (my higher self) speaking to me, part of my energy that's back there (between lives), speaking to me in Latin.

And those words…?
"Vanum populatum."

Does the meaning of that deepen now that you…?
They're all amused by the cleverness of me speaking to me in Latin to myself, knowing I (in this life) don't speak Latin, never studied Latin, would write it down because it was unusual, and then knowing I would look it up (on the internet) and find the Latin translation. Knowing that only by my forcing myself to examine these words as a puzzle, would I come to embrace or understand them. As if just saying "Destroy the Ego," or "Annihilate Vanity" wouldn't help me get it - I had to Google it in order to understand it. And knowing the concept was the same I'd learned in Tibetan philosophy about stripping away the ego. What they're saying to me is "If you heard it as a phrase you would have dismissed it, but because you heard it in another language, you gave it depth."

Had to dwell on it.
They're showing me a past life I had in Rome. I was a patrician, a teacher of Latin and Ethics. I can feel the feeling of the toga around me as I walk, and as I reach into my pocket, I can feel the sensation of what Roman era coins felt like to my touch. I'm stopping at a food stand in Pompeii, being greeted by others, and nodding to them. I didn't die in the eruption - actually there had been some kind of scandal with me and a slave, something about me spending more time with my slaves because they were much more entertaining and educated in a different way and that somehow brought shame to my family. My wife's family - I think it's her father and brother, who supplied the poison - so that she would live on in the style and luxury to which she was accustomed. But I had true friendship here - especially with these people who were considered my slaves; I considered them my teachers.

Even though I was rather successful and wealthy from teaching Ethics, it was a fun and unusual life. Ah, okay, in my current life in film, I've written a story about a character living in Rome during this era; they're showing me that my past lives parallel my writing…

Ok. Let me ask another of question… I'm asking them about a project I'm working on right now, and the question I'm asking them is, "Is this important?" and they're hesitant to respond, in the desire to not direct me where I may already be going.. They enjoy saying to me "You know the answer, why are you bothering us with the question?" But the answer is -- that this person I'm writing about had a tremendous amount of influence, energy-wise, on the planet, and that's why it's important to tell the story, or work on the story, or even recreate the story in a writer's mind. Whether it gets made or not is not important, but the focus on the person and the energy is... Okay I get that.[28]

It makes sense to you...
Yes. My next question is about my family. I already know the answer; my wife is what someone might call an angel -- a spirit that is selfless and loving, and knows I need grounding. And my daughter is yes, a very old soul... as I knew. And my son is the same, a little younger soul, but as playful as me.

NOTE: At some point the lead member of my council said "Richard already knows the answer to this question," and an image appeared before me of myself on the couch, with Jimmy Quast sitting next to me. That image and answer made me realize he was addressing my eternal presence, or spirit – and by saying "Richard" he was referring to the guy on the couch – my present incarnation.

A QUESTION ABOUT THE LIFE ESSENCE

The specific question I have is when my daughter Olivia was born, I had this vision of men dressed in white; older men with beards, surrounding her. She was only a few days old lying in the bed next to me, and I was completely aware of their presence.

I'm asking them about this, how there was one elderly man standing in the center of this semicircle around the little baby Olivia - and he was pouring something into her body from a copper vase, like an antique funnel -- as he was pouring this golden liquid out of the funnel I panicked and shouted "What are you doing?" He turned around and said simply; "This is how it's done." So I'm asking (the council) about "What was the liquid?" (Pause) Uh... nobody wants to fess up.

(Pause, as I understood their answer) Ok, what I saw as a liquid -- it was energy... I want to say, I'm not sure if I should reveal this to you, but it's a little bit of predetermination of how long a person might be on the planet.

For her?
For everyone. When you're born, there's this little bit of a determination of how much energy you will have and I was seeing a demonstration of filling a person up with that... or maybe they're teasing me with this answer. I can't tell. They are letting me ramble on with this story and are not talking. Maybe I'm not supposed to reveal this information. I can't tell; they do that.

---

[28] I wound up working on "Amelia," starring Hilary Swank, and assisting them with all of their research into Earhart's life before she disappeared.

This is separate and apart from her soul energy committed to her life?
Separate and apart from her spirit, but it was like visualization of what your life experiences are. I mean it was like literally coming out as a golden liquid into a funnel into her, and everyone in the vision looked at me like, "Why are you asking this question? This is obvious." I'm not getting a straight answer (from the council) from anybody... They're all just saying... not it's "none of your business," but it's something you'll figure out eventually.

You had a question about music?
Music, well that was answered. [29]

(Refers to the list of questions) What about your friend Paul and your dad?
Paul, is a young soul. Dad, a bit older soul. Just a great guy, both great people. Paul's very... like me, sense of humor; he's saying his excuse is that he's younger and he's working stuff out... [30]

What color is he?
White.

Your dad?
Golden, more yellow. Little twinge of orange, maybe that's the architect in him. But Paul's a young soul, I was very angry with him for dying early, dying young...

Can you understand it was by plan?
Oh yeah, it's true.

Does that mean they didn't pour enough of that stuff into him?
(Chuckles) Or he mistook it for a beer, which is one of the difficult issues he spent a part his life working on. (Pause) They're telling me "You already know the answer to whatever question you have, just meditate on it, and go within, and the answer will come to you." Also "keep up the good work."[31]

Anything from them about Wa' tanka?
I healed and touched a lot of people. The reverberation from that is important. I was able to do that in difficult circumstances, but by and large, a happy circumstance... somehow I turn what seems difficult into a happy circumstance; a bit more fun.

---

[29] Meaning: the idea of energy transfer and why I chose to learn different musical instruments, and how my lifelong connection to music has to do with the transmission of the energy.
[30] In my mind's eye, I see my father as a young man in his 40's, and standing next to him, my friend Paul, looking as I knew him in his 20's, but am feeling more like he's a brother, than a friend.
[31] These questions I'd wondered about, and by meditating on them had come to various conclusions prior to the session.

So even though the other tribe...
Goddamned Hurons.

Damned Hurons... (Laughs)
I don't see it as a predetermined, before life agreement;[32] the tribe had issues they were working on, and there was an ego dispute between a Chief of the Huron and the Chief of our tribe. I know there are other names for our tribe (Lakota) but we just refer to ourselves as The People.[33] Ultimately the battle between us was more about a war of insults, tit for tat - revenge.

NOTE: As I remembered, the arguments, war council, planning for battle came back to me in a flash.

NOTHING IS PREDETERMINED

And they went beyond the plan a bit, or a lot?
Honestly, everybody was in agreement; "Eh, when you act out of revenge, this is what happens." People get hacked up if you don't find a way to resolve your differences. There is always the opportunity to change the contract, or the path. You can always change your so called 'karma,' if you resolve to change.

There's nothing predetermined. You don't have to pick up the rifle to kill someone, even if that's part of your contract or your reason to be on the planet. You can always learn, change, and evolve. You don't have to go through a whole lifetime to learn one lesson.

It's just that simple, isn't it?
(Resisting agreeing) It's very difficult. Because even after you've made an agreement to live a particular life or act in a particular way to help yourself and others, you can change the agreement - if you can find the determination within yourself to change yourself and those around you and put your energy towards curing and healing.

Simple to say, but difficult to do.
Very difficult. And when you see the agreement going awry, it's sort of "Well, we did agree upon this and we didn't get to the point we should have." In my mind, you haven't worked hard enough to change the dynamic in a healing way. That's my feeling. But I'm unusual that way. (Laughs) Not everybody (in this realm) agrees with my point of view.

Anyone else you'd like to see?
(As I'm heading back, I see my father, handsome, young, in his 40's, standing next to my friend Paul Tracey, in his early 20's - side by side, happy to see me. I stop

[32] Meaning the killing of my tribe by the Huron tribe with regard to the testimony that sometimes people who kill each other do it as part of an agreement to learn something deeper.
[33] I didn't know this, but it is accurate. "The Sioux: Life and Customs" by Royal Hassrick pg 73

to kiss my father on the head.) I'm just giving a loving kiss on the forehead to my father. Thanking him. (Laughs) "Get back to work." That's what he said.

Anything else you'd like to impart to Rich?
To tell him he needs to try to be more in the moment, in the present, and just... let... go.

Remember these experiences you've had, you're not alone, and you have a big bunch of friends.
(Pause) Hmm. I'm just saying goodbye to everybody. They say "See you later." I ask "When?" They all laugh; they're not about to tell me. (Chuckles) Very funny. Okay.

Remember this world is always with you and within you... and you may have moments of clarity in the days ahead, all is retained to help and empower you with renewed energy and greater... What was it?
Patience.

Back through the tunnel to the present as I count from one to ten... back to a very fortunate life."
In the first class I visited during my session, everyone welcomed me as if the Teacher's Pal had arrived. In Luana's class however, the teacher stopped speaking, the class turned as if to say "Why are you here?" The students mocked my simplistic description of their complex work. Apparently not everyone can get attend this advanced class. Somehow I'd found a hall pass to get in.

Recently I was at a family funeral in upper Wisconsin. I happened to speak to a relative who is a Lakota Sioux historian, something I was unaware of. I said "I had this unusual vision while under hypnosis about me being what I appeared to be a Lakota." He stopped me. "How many feathers did you have and were they up or down?" I said, "Two, they were down." He said "That means you were a medicine man. What did they call you?" I said "Sounded like Watanka." He said "Wakantanka or Wa'tanka means The Great Spirit, and what they call medicine men." I said "If that's true, then why would I think the Huron killed my tribe when they're located on the East Coast?" He said, "We're actually sitting near a spot they fought over for 60 years in Eau Claire, Wisconsin." He confirmed details that I tried to confirm on my own but couldn't.

In my session, I met my spirit guide, who seemed to be someone I've known forever, and then found my soul group of fellow travelers. I visited classrooms where I got to see myself through other's eyes. I'd made a trip to my council where they confirmed a number of details about my life that seemed extraordinary. I had the same experience Newton's clients had. And most improbably of all, I felt as if I'd gone to the classroom Luana had told me about before her passing – I saw her there, spoke to her, felt as if I'd really seen and heard from my dear departed friend.

I felt as if the Earth had suddenly shifted on its axis. Everything I thought I knew about the planet, about humanity, about *life*, had been altered by this session.

My skeptical, conscious mind kept hammering at this new information. Had I really just seen a past life? Was I just eager to make it up? How would that account for details I didn't know until later? Or could it be I'd already been through this psychic door, and like most people, merely ignored the signs and messages that had already come from the Great Beyond?

I cannot think of permanent enmity between man and man, and believing as I do in the theory of reincarnation, I live in the hope that if not in this birth, in some other birth I shall be able to hug all of humanity in friendly embrace.

- Mahatma Gandhi

CHAPTER 8
I HEAR DEAD PEOPLE

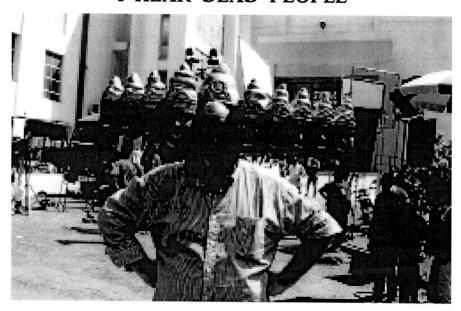

If it's the Psychic Network why do they need a phone number?

- Robin Williams

I once awoke to see a man with a noose around his neck dangling in the stairway. I gasped. The man in the noose looked up, took it off, and then scrambled down a ladder. In an Aussie accent he said "I'm terribly sorry, mate, it's just something I feel the need to do." I was staying at filmmakers Phillip Noyce and Jan Sharp's home in Sydney, Australia. They'd recently sold their home but there was a window before it went off the market, and I was invited to stay in the nearly empty house. I was startled to awake to this vision of a hanging man. I learned from Jan that a painter of the house had hanged himself some years earlier.

"I hear dead people," to paraphrase the line from "The Sixth Sense."[34] Every now and then I hear from the dead, or imagine I do. It's entirely plausible the part of my brain that retains voice memory is accessed and like a schizophrenic, as in Ron Howard's "Beautiful Mind," I hear voices that don't exist.

Some years after Luana passed, I was staying at an apartment near NYU when I thought I heard Luana speaking to me. In this half-awake state she told me I needed to find her friend Vic Ramos; he needed help. Vic managed Matt Dillon and other actors, and some years after she passed, he asked me to bring some of Luana's ashes to his magnificent roof garden overlooking Manhattan. But I couldn't remember his address, and couldn't track it down. A few weeks later I learned Vic caught pneumonia the night I heard from Luana; he'd gone into the hospital and died suddenly.[35]

I was invited to London by an author, Nigel Spence, who wanted me to adapt a novel he'd written. He lives in a centuries old building and had me stay in his office, an old room he's adapted into a loft. The first night there, I awoke to find myself sitting in a room of soldiers. As I looked around, they were all looking at me, grinning, as if to say "Look what the cat dragged in." I asked who they were. They said they worked for The King, and rounded up people who didn't pay taxes, or did naughty things. I didn't feel any particular fear on my part; they seemed like a happy gang of men dressed in what appeared to be 18th century armor.

The following morning I asked Nigel about the history of the house. "It was an old building that was owned in the 18th century by the Royal family. Some kind of police station is what I've been told." It was a dream, but an odd one methinks.

Another incident involved a musician friend who lives in France. He and I had played some blues together in the wee hours at a club in Monte Carlo, and I spent the night on the couch in his chateau. I was awoken by a person with an English accent saying "Who the *f**k* are you?" I was startled, and looked around the living room, but didn't see anyone. I recognized the voice; it was my friend's father, a famous musician who died some years earlier. I said something like "I'm a friend of your son's, and just spending the night on his couch." That seemed to mollify

[34] Written by M. Night Shyamalan
[35] I have a small framed photograph of Luana and Vic on my desk, which was given to me by his assistant who told me it was his favorite, and sat on his desk. They're holding arms around each other and grinning - as I'm sure they're doing as I write this sentence.

him - I never mentioned to my friend that it seemed his dad was keeping an eye on his son's house guests.

I was teaching at The Workshops in Camden, Maine and was staying at the new extension they'd built next to the campus. One morning I awoke to find a Mohican Indian at the end of my bed. Shaved scalp, a knife in one hand, and a small axe in the other, red paint, or blood, all over his body. He was screaming at me at the top of his lungs in a language I didn't understand, but took to mean "GET OUT!!!!" After gasping and seeing him dissolve before my eyes, I put up my hands and said "Dude. You gotta relax. I'm only here for a couple of days, and then I'll be long gone."

This vision wasn't a dream, as I was sitting up in bed, eyes open when I saw him. He was as clear as anything I've ever seen, blood dripping from his axe and the knife in his hands, his veins bulging as he screamed at me. Not exactly a welcoming committee to my first day of teaching; I didn't stay there again.

But what is the mechanism for ghosts? This research says that once we're off the earthly plane, we're "outside of time." The choice to hang around a favorite haunt, like a barfly who won't leave, isn't hard to do, or an unfathomable task. Reports say that at some point the ghost's spirit guide shows up and says something to the effect of, "Don't you think it's time to head home?" It's the ghostly equivalent of "You don't have to go home, but you can't stay here." Perhaps the ghost is traumatized – if they can't decide to leave, the compassionate thing to do seems to be to guide them "into the light," and suggest perhaps it's time to call a taxi and journey home.

I've seen two ghosts in Santa Monica; the first was in The Sea Castle, a large building built by Charlie Chaplin in the 1930's overlooking the ocean. I was sleeping on the couch in a friend's apartment when I awoke to see a pretty blond girl with long hair, crying on the couch. When I blinked, she disappeared. Later, I said to my friend, "Who's the ghost in your apartment?" He blanched. He'd taken over the apartment from a friend whose girlfriend had committed suicide in that very room. The daughter of that woman, whom I later met, looked exactly like the blond I saw crying on the couch.

I was living in a bungalow built in the 1930's when I'd wake up because it felt like someone had sat down on my bed. Finally, in a dream state, I pictured a male in his 30's, who would sit down on the bed and watch me sleep. One night I felt him climb into bed with me; that was the last straw. I said out loud; "Look, Ghost, I have no problem with you hanging around my apartment, but you are *not allowed in the bed!*" That seemed to work, and he didn't bother me again.

One morning the new tenant from the apartment next door came screaming into my bungalow. She said she was brushing her teeth when she looked up in the mirror and saw a man standing behind her. When she turned, he disappeared. I said "Oh, is he about 30, brown hair?" She nodded. I said "He's the resident ghost. Just tell him not to bother you."

There are other stories of visitations I've heard about from my relatives; my cousin Marcus had a strong sensation he should drive over to our grandfather Valentino's house the day he died. Later, Marcus was given the old leather chair Valentino sat in night after night in his living room. Marcus was downstairs in his darkroom developing some photographs, when he emerged to see our grandfather sitting in the leather chair, smoking a cigar and smiling at him. Marcus was so startled he backed up, and closed the door of the darkroom. He said he opened the door "And papa was still there." Marcus ran up the stairs from the basement, and I was the first person he told this story to.

His mother had a visitation as well; Elma said when her husband Tom died after a long illness, he appeared at the end of her bed looking as healthy as the day she met him. He said "I'm fine. I love you Elma." A split second later, the phone rang; the hospital called to say that he'd passed.

I was chatting with my skeptical dentist about my reincarnation film. (Mouth agape, him bemused) He said "I don't believe in that crap." Then he said, "But I had a patient who was a psychic and one day she said something unusual to me. My father had died recently and my mother was debating whether to throw out his old shoes. I told her to get rid of them. But while working on this psychic, she suddenly said, "Your father wants you to keep the shoes.""

A prolific television producer told me his mother recently had a visitation from his father. His mother moved to Florida after his father's passing, and one night, as she lying in bed reading, her husband appeared, walked past her, went over to his side of the bed and climbed in. He looked at her and said simply "I just wanted to see if you're all right," and disappeared. My friends' mother said to him, "I've never believed in ESP or any version of the afterlife. But after seeing my husband sitting next to me, I'm convinced there's something to it."

The energy that we contain during our lifetime doesn't disappear, it appears to travel to a place that it came from, and rejoin the others that it's always known. However, we're also connected to the other energy forms we've known through our lifetime, and returning to visit with them may be difficult, but it's akin to the magic of picking up a cell phone on one side of the planet, and getting an answer.

But if spirits can decide to stick around after they've departed, then how does that account for other phenomena that aren't related to ghosts?

While in D.C, I was walking by the reflecting pond in front of the Lincoln memorial. Suddenly I was overcome by an intense feeling of sadness, tears coming to my eyes. I realized I was walking past the Vietnam War memorial. I don't know anyone who died in Vietnam, yet if I walked a few feet past the panel of names, the feeling disappeared. I walked back; it returned. I returned years later with a video camera, and the same emotion arose at the same panel.

Since no ghosts are there, perhaps the memorial is a place where people deposit their sadness. Perhaps that particular panel is one many people had put the energy of their sadness over the loss of a beloved. Is marble more conducive to retaining energy than stone? I have no idea, but the feeling was palpable.

I had a similar experience visiting Anne Frank's house in Amsterdam. I'd read and seen "The Diary Of Anne Frank," and when climbing the steep steps the layout of her hiding place came rushing back to me. The fake door they used to enter their home, the steep steps to get up into the attic, the room where Anne talked about seeing the neighbor's tree in the back yard next door.

As I entered the room where various editions of her book are on display, I was hit by an overwhelming wave of sadness. I looked around the room to see what specifically had caught my eye to bring on this feeling. There were only panels of pages of the book written in various languages, and letters from people around the world who had been touched by her story. When I stepped out of the room, the feeling disappeared. As I stepped back in, the wave hit me again. Could it be possible people who visited this place had somehow deposited a certain amount of the energy that we call "sadness?"

The third place was the Book Depository in Dallas from where JFK was reportedly shot. I felt a creeping sensation of energy that brings on melancholy and intense sadness. I spoke to a guard about it, asking him if he'd ever felt an odd energy in that room. "Oh yeah," he said. "There's some kind of deep sadness about this place, and I can feel it from time to time."

Is it possible for someone to deposit energy into an object? A marble memorial? A room full of books? If so, then what is the mechanism involved? People say sometimes that they can "feel" the presence of a loved one through a favorite object, a watch, or in the case of my grandfather, his favorite leather chair. But is this energy transference quantifiable?

Here's a story of the energy of a book, courtesy of Eric Davis of the "Movie Phone" blog. Anthony Hopkins (who once told me he loved Luana's acting) starred in 'The Girl from Petrovka,' based on a book by George Feifer. After signing on for the film, he reportedly tried to track down a copy of the book while in London but couldn't find one. He entered the Leicester Square stop to board a train when he spotted a copy of 'The Girl from Petrovka' on a nearby bench.

"Two years later while filming in Vienna, author George Feifer visited the set. During a conversation with Hopkins, Feifer mentioned he didn't have a copy of his own book -- he'd lent his last one (complete with his own annotations) to a friend who had lost it somewhere in London. Hopkins, puzzled, then fetched his copy, which also had notes in the margins. When he showed it to Feifer, the author confirmed that, amazingly, it was the same book."

I first became familiar with the term "out of body experience" through the writings of Robert Monroe. Monroe's books are about "astral projection," the sensation of being able to visit other places on the planet while "out of body." Monroe gives a blow by blow description of how to effectively take oneself on an out of body journey, the feeling of the etheric body rising up out of the material body and floating around the room. He catalogues the times he did so and details sessions when he traveled to visit someone, pinched or tickled them, and then confirmed later they'd felt his pinch.[36]

This is a controversial and subjective subject, for if a person has never had an out of body experience it's a bit like explaining what it's like to be drunk. It's hard to describe the numbness and sensations that accompany a trip down that particular lane to someone who's never touched alcohol.

I've had them a few times, and once while visiting my Italian relatives in the Alps. I was awoken by three spirits hovering nearby and they invited me to come with them. I felt myself rise up and out of my body and start to zoom through the atmosphere. But not knowing anything about this research, and quite startled by it, I stopped and turned around. "I don't think I'm supposed to go here yet." Little did I know what an adventure it might have been.

I met a young girl from Iceland living in Florence during my Junior Year Abroad in Rome, and some 20 years after we met got the chance to see her and her son in Halmstad, Sweden. She introduced me to her brother, who told me he was a "psychic healer." I asked him how he'd come to his occupation.

He'd been in a motorcycle accident and his leg wouldn't heal and as a result wasn't able to work. He began to pray for help from his relatives, as he explained to me that Icelanders, instead of praying to a particular God, pray to their deceased relatives to intercede on their behalf.

He claimed one night he woke to see a spirit in his room, operating on his leg. A man was standing over him, his hands inside of his leg, and somehow fixing his broken leg. He said when he awoke, his leg had healed. But there were complications that ensued, as if some kind of door to the outside world had been opened, and unusual psychic events began to happen. At night, spirits would show up unannounced, and once he and his wife one night awoke to find the bed shaking and levitating.

It was unnerving for his wife, to say the least, and she left him. At that point, he said men "dressed in white" began showing up in his room. At first they'd take his hand, help him out of his body and he'd "fly around the room" as an astral projection. He said this continued for an entire summer and couldn't remember where they would take him. Eventually, he started to become conscious of the journey and realized they'd fly over a great distance to a place where they taught him about spiritual healing. The lessons he learned there he'd brought back, which he was using by working as a healer with patients in Sweden.

This was many years before I'd heard of classes in the afterlife, and seeing an opportunity to learn something without having to go through the same trauma, I asked him to describe what these "spirit guides" had taught him.

---

[36] Robert Monroe's work on OBE's is listed in the bibliography.

He said they taught him to picture his clients sitting in the "bright healing light of the universe." He'd meditate on their illness, and if it existed in some particular place, a shoulder perhaps, or a leg, and he'd focus the light onto the place where they had pain and use the light to heal them. He said the light came from somewhere deep in the Universe, and was a bright white healing light, and that his lessons had been in learning how to focus this healing light.

It wasn't until I ran across Michael Newton that I started to read of other people who'd been approached by "men dressed in white," for lessons from people in the afterlife. It also coincided with Luana's recurring dream of a classroom with people "dressed in white" who were being given lessons about healing. Either people were making this up on different continents to different people, or they were having some kind of shared experience with this "healing energy."

But what is it? Is it an energy that can be identified?

Apparently, between lives many of us attend classes in energy transfer and healing. I asked a woman why she named her daughter Krystal, and she said "I've never told anyone, but I had this recurring dream about speaking to an elderly man dressed in white in a cave of crystal." I told her a bit about this research and she elaborated on her vision, "Sometimes I'm in a classroom with people dressed in white, and the teacher writes formulas on a type of board. When he's through writing the formula, the object appears, spinning in front of him. The object is geometric in shape, is made of energy and makes the sound of icicles melting."

In the chapter in this book called "Aquaphobia," Sophia says that energy packets follow us through life carrying bits of our past lives. In the chapter "Vanum Populatum," I say I attended a class where geometric shapes that carry our past life energy come to be replenished and "cleaned." This energy appears to be born of the essence of the universe, composed of some quantifiable amount of energy that exists in each of us. Further, science tells us energy can't be destroyed and has a tendency to seek out other energy patterns it was previously affiliated with. In like form it appears this spirit energy seeks out souls or energy groups it's been affiliated with before. Could this be "dark matter" that quantum physics speaks of? Could it be the ether that connects and bonds the universe?

Upon our return to Earth, it's just a matter of time before others in our energy or soul group, like errant ions, will seek us out. It appears to be no coincidence you've known your best friend forever. You have. In his book "Linked: How Everything Is Connected to Everything Else and What It Means" noted scientist Albert-László Barabási shows how social networks mirror nature in how many people orbit around us at a given time. We congregate in packs, the way atoms congregate and seek each other out. His description of pods of friends, mirrors Michael Newton's research on "soul groups" in the afterlife.

The energy of the spirit world appears to be ever present in our world, we can access it if need be, access the energy that was once here which appears to us as apparitions or ghosts.[37] The energy that psychics tap into is a quantifiable energy closely related to the energy spoken of in quantum physics. Our ability to connect to it is the same as encountering gravity on a daily basis - we can't see the energy that pulls the apple from the tree to the ground, but we know it's there, and we use it to navigate our world.

Another unusual energy event that happens in everyday lives is "déjà vu." We're walking in a place, or moving through a space, and we suddenly get the feeling we've experienced this event before. In my case, I've had déjà vu events - one in particular included the Italian film director Lina Wertmuller.

Lina Wertmuller worked for Federico Fellini as an Art Director, and later directed some classic Italian films. In 1975, I was going to school in Rome when I had a dream about her. I told my friends about it; I saw her standing in an elevator wearing her distinctive white glasses. I had no idea why I would dream about seeing her in an elevator. Two years later, I found myself living in San Francisco, selling stereo equipment. While living in the city in 1977, I read in Herb Caen's column that Lina was in town making a feature film. And I remembered the dream I'd had, and wondered if it was possible to interview her. I'd written a freelance article for the Italian American magazine "Identity" and I queried the editor. They were more interested in an interview with Giancarlo Giannini, who was starring in the film.

I booked myself a room in the same hotel they were staying in, then introduced myself to someone on the crew, and asked about interviewing the famous actor, who'd starred in "Seven Beauties" "The Seduction of Mimi" and other classic Wertmuller films.

One night I got a call from Giannini; he came over to my room with a bottle of wine, and proceeded to regale me with hilarious stories of his life growing up in Rome. I think we might have polished off two bottles that night, as I remember getting an early call the next morning that startled me out of bed; Giancarlo wanted me to come down to breakfast, as he had a couple of more things he wanted to impart. And as I rode in the elevator downstairs, the door opened, and there was Lina Wertmuller, exactly as I'd seen her in my dream; wearing white rimmed glasses, a white outfit, on her way to the set. I had a buzzing sensation in my head, as I wasn't quite awake yet, and it felt like I was in a dream, exactly the way I felt when I'd had the dream. I didn't speak to her, as I was dumbstruck at reliving a moment that I'd dreamt of, at least two years previously.

There was also a time when I saw a ghost of a person who hadn't passed away. My first visit to Dharamsala, India, I attended a dinner for The State Oracle of Tibet. A young man with a smile that lights up the room, Thupten Ngodrup became the Nechung Kuten, or the "Medium of the State Oracle of Tibet" under unusual circumstances. Oracles have a long history in Tibet, and like the Oracle

---

[37] Michael Talbot's "The Holographic Universe," speaks of quantum physics and wave particle theory, and how it may be that all experiences are stored in a holographic manner - the actual light waves that capture events never disappear, and can be accessed the way a piece of a hologram contains its entire contents.

of Delphi, leaders would go to them for advice on any number of things. The previous Oracle had magically guided the 14th Dalai Lama out of Tibet just in time to save him from the Chinese taking him hostage.[38] That Oracle passed away in 1984, and the Nechung Monastery did pujas, or prayer sessions for the next three years, trying to gain guidance for whomever would become the next Oracle.

In the midst of one prayer session, a young Nechung monk fell down and went into a seizure. When he woke up, everyone was staring at him. Apparently he'd been speaking in an ancient Tibetan language and cursing out those around him. The young monk went through a series of rigorous tests, and eventually, the Dalai Lama declared Thubten the new Nechung Oracle, affectionately called "Kutenla."

I've been able to witness the Oracle during one of his sessions and it's unusual. For about an hour, the Nechung monks do a series of prayers and play instruments to put him into the mindset required for his trance. At some point, he blacks out, and his attendants put a 60 pound headdress on him, tightly strapping it down. When his eyes open, he starts to hiss and growl, and leaps up, as if trying to escape. Sometimes he pulls out swords and twirls them in elaborate movements that would be lethal in an amateur's hands, and eventually his attendants grab hold of him and strap him into a chair. He begins to speak in an ancient dialect, (they consider the voice to be that of an ancient Tibetan warrior named Dorje Drakden) and his attendants write down the advice he gives.

I asked him what he remembered during a session, and he said it's like having a dream. The headdress is incredibly heavy, I noticed that Kutenla's upper shoulders are not the kind you'd find on a man who can spin with a 60 pound weight on their head for an hour. During his session, I noticed that his tongue turned black, and the very shape of his face appeared different. It might have been the stress of wearing the headdress, but it is unusual to say the least.

While visiting Kutenla in India, he asked if I was interested in filming interviews with 150 young refugees who'd arrived from Tibet. I followed them as they learned about life in the west and met the Dalai Lama for the first time. I heard amazing stories from these children and teens, some of them monks and nuns who were tortured in Tibet, telling stories of how they'd escaped, or were forced out, and their incredible journeys to freedom.[39] Many were young children, sent by their parents to learn about their culture and language, never to see their parents again. Oddly, while interviewing them, I had the feeling my trip had been pre-ordained so I could allow these people to tell their story on camera.

But after my visit to Dharamsala, Kutenla came to visit Los Angeles. I gave him a tour which included Paramount studios ("Over here, reality; over there, unreality") and The Getty Museum. We stopped by my place in Santa Monica, where he offered to say a prayer, and blessed my abode. The hilarious and generous Goldie

---

[38] This scene famous depicted in Martin Scorsese's "Kundun."

[39] The documentary can be found on youtube as "Tibetan Refugee Part One."

Hawn organized a dinner for him at her and Kurt Russell's home in the Pacific Palisades, and Kutenla and his attendant monks were guests. I was exhausted, and when Kutenla invited me to come with him to Disneyland the next day, I declined. I was just too pooped to keep up the pace.

That night, as I was sleeping in my place in Santa Monica, I heard a knock at the door. I got up to answer it, and there standing in the hallway, glowing from head to toe, was Kutenla. I realized I was in a dream, but it was unlike any dream I'd had. "My I come in?" he asked. "Certainly," I said. "You're always welcome in my home." He came in and looked around, then smiled. "You know, I would really appreciate it if you came to Disneyland with me tomorrow." I laughed. What a wonderful way to be able to reconsider a position. "I'd be honored."

The next morning, I was awoken by a phone call, and it was Kutenla's attendant Tenzing calling. "Richard-la, the Oracle thinks he might have left his camera bag in your car and perhaps you could drive to Disneyland to deliver it to him?" I said "Please tell him I got his message in my dream last night, and I will join you."

We had an enjoyable day at the "Happiest Place on Earth." Everywhere we went, people assumed these Tibetan monks were part of another ride, along with Goofy and Snow White. I told him the dream I had the night before; he didn't have a clue as to what I was referring to. If he *had* visited me, it was purely in spirit form; his conscious mind was not aware of it.

Finally, ghost visits must run in my family; both my children have had them. Recently Olivia and her mom went to the funeral of a respected Los Angeles attorney my wife worked for.[40] At the funeral, while someone was on the altar of the Church extolling the virtues of the deceased, Olivia said "Look mom, he's up there," and pointed as if she saw him flying above. Sherry said "Why is he here?" Olivia said, "He's smiling. He likes this." She then saw him standing on the altar, just behind his beloved friends who'd come to sing his praises. (Yes, despite being an attorney).

One day my son RJ said he didn't want to go upstairs. I asked why, and he said "There's a lady up there." I asked him who it was, and he walked me into the kitchen and pointed to a photo of Luana on the fridge. "Luana's upstairs?" I asked. He nodded. "Well, does she frighten you?" I asked. With his hands out, he said "Dad! You can see right through her!" I saw his point. Someone you can look through might be disconcerting to a three year old. I asked, "Does she say anything to you?" He thought about it. "She says "I love you R.J." He looked up at me with his huge hazel eyes. He was serious, and I wanted to assuage his fears. I said, "Well that doesn't sound very scary." He sighed. "Okaaay," he said, and headed upstairs.

One day my wife Sherry was looking at a painting that Luana had painted before she passed away. It was unusual, featuring a portrait of a woman and a man, but the two were melding into one another. She thought "I wonder who that man in the

---

[40] "Robert Berke, Activist Attorney" LA Times 12-3-2009

painting is?" He had a moustache and looked Latin. An hour later she was walking on Santa Monica beach and a handsome older man approached and complimented her on her hair. They started to speak, and he revealed that he was Gene Shacove, the famous Beverly Hills hairdresser, and revealed that the movie "Shampoo" was about his salon.

Sherry asked if he knew Luana – of course he did, as the screenwriter Robert Towne was a close friend – in fact Luana's tempestuous relationship with a Latin Casanova hairdresser named Richard Alcala was the basis for Robert's script. After Sherry asked him about the painting, Gene said, "I can tell you who the man is in that painting. It's Richard, and he and Luana dated back in the 1960's."

Coincidence? How could it be that Sherry would ask a question of a painting, and an hour later be led to the answer in this unlikely manner? This research shows that what appears coincidental, may in fact have purpose.

But in order for this research to truly bear fruit, I needed to interview a past life regressionist who'd had similar results, but who'd never heard of life between life sessions or Michael Newton. One came to me out of the blue.

"After all, it is no more surprising to be born twice than it is to be born once."

- Voltaire

CHAPTER 9
I'VE GOT A GIFT FOR YOU

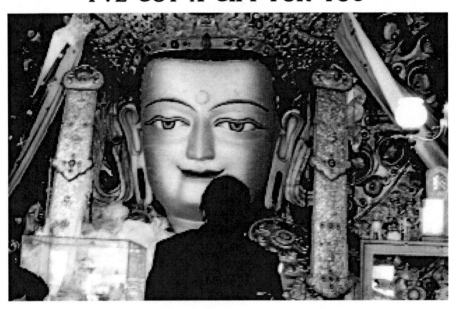

"So as through a glass and darkly, the age long strife I see, Where I fought in many guises, many names, but always me."

- General George S. Patton

But what about people who've had similar experiences, but have never heard of this form or research? I got a call from my friend Dr. Habib Sadeghi. A successful holistic Doctor practicing in West Los Angeles,[41] we'd crossed paths and became instant friends. We'd spend hours discussing Tibetan medicine, or what I'd been learning in this research and how it might apply to modern medicine. He called me one day to introduce his friend Debbie Haynie, a therapist from Denver.

Debbie[42] is a psychotherapist and healer, dedicated to the integration of the body, mind and spirit/soul. She's never heard of "Life between Lives" therapy or the research behind it.

INTERVIEW WITH DEBBIE HAYNIE

RM: Tell me what you do, please.
DH: I have a psycho-spiritual practice in Denver, Colorado. The psycho-spiritual practice focuses on integration of the body, mind and spirit. In the realm of my work, I do anything from hypnosis to shamanic work, the old indigenous medicine ways, helping people to connect more with who they are. I've been working in this field for 27 years, graduating eventually into the spirit realm, and most of my calling to this work came from spirit and some of my own experiences.

Could you talk about some of the clients you've worked with and some of the experiences they've had with past life regressions?
One of the realms of past life regression I explore is the arena where we look at health issues, injuries, pains in the body that don't make any sense in the medical world. My favorite story is about a woman I worked with who was from the corporate world. She was in a position of responsibility for many people in a large corporation, and there was a reorganization going on; she felt extremely sad about so many people being laid off. She had developed an excruciating pain in her right arm, and went from specialist to specialist but they couldn't find any reason for her pain. So we scheduled a past life regression and she went back to a lifetime in the 1300's when she was in a battle. She was a man in that lifetime, the head of a group of men she led into this battle. She had anticipated fewer men on the other side of their battle, and they were overtaken and the entire group had been killed.

Upon her death we found her lying on the ground with the sword in her hand, tightly held, and her last thoughts (which we often talk about in past life regression, what are those last thoughts that you had just prior to your death), was "I'm responsible for these people, what am I going to do now? I'm responsible for them, and they're all dead." I helped her remove the sword and we brought some healing to that part of her that existed in that life and had her repeat new thoughts; "It's not my fault, I'm not responsible for other people's suffering," and the pain went away.

---

[41] Behiveofhealing.com

[42] www.antaskarana.com

She brought the stress and psychic memory of that past life into this one when faced with a similar situation; all she needed to do was acknowledge that fact.

PAST LIFE THERAPY FOR CHILDREN

Have you had any experience doing past life regression with children?
Some of the other work I do is with children's past lives, because for them the veil between worlds is so thin, often times they can clearly remember them. One example is a five year old boy who was having extreme social problems on the playground. He was hitting other kids, throwing rocks at them, acting really aggressive. He had been taken to all the traditional modalities; a psychiatrist, a psychologist, a pediatrician and no one could really figure out what was wrong. The Doctors wanted to put him on medication, which his parents didn't want to do, and was part of the reason they brought him to me.

With children, you do past life work a little bit differently, and he pretty clearly remembered a previous lifetime of slavery and remembered the physical act of being tarred and feathered. And so we healed that part of him, helping him eliminate the fears connected with that trauma. Interestingly enough, from that point on, the aggression immediately stopped. The Pediatrician couldn't believe that his behavior had shifted so dramatically. He is now eleven years old and doing really well.

I think the implications are that sometimes we bring past memories of trauma with us into this life, and we can see those manifest in some children. The strong memory of a trauma from a previous life can wind up creating developmental problems in those children.

Even if people don't believe in past life regressions, this work can help various individuals, because sometimes people have psychosomatic symptoms and psychological symptoms that manifest in their daily lives. When we do this type of work, we're bringing someone into a sort of energetic field, and then help those things that need to shift within the body or the psyche. The shifting occurs in areas traditional psychological methods sometimes cannot access, or medical methods can affect. Even if you're not a believer, these memories may be used as a metaphor, and how they might affect aspects of your life. The process can help shift and change some of our beliefs as well as heal our minds.

SOUL MATES

Have you had any past life love stories that needed resolution in this life?
One of the interesting topics in this work is obsession; someone a person is infatuated with, or in love with, and why they're so attracted to them. In past life regressions we get a chance to examine arenas involving the heart and why we choose people we wind up with romantically - for good reasons or bad ones. There

was a particular woman I worked with, who dealt with these issues.

She was from the Corporate world; under normal circumstances very logical, and in the beginning didn't believe in past life regression at all. She'd met a married man at a particular conference and was immediately drawn to him. For a year they had this torrid, intense relationship. She felt very connected, very alive - 'soul-mate' type of material. But he chose not to continue the relationship, and went back to his wife and family. She was devastated and went into a severe depression. We decided she would try a past life regression to see whether they had met in a previous life.

It turned out there was a lifetime in England where they lived on a farm. It was one of those lifetimes that was very happy, an enjoyable one to go back to. However, she had a son already in this marriage (who in her present life is also her son, which is a form of reunion, someone who's come back into our life in a lovely way) and pregnant with a second child. It was premature and tragically she died giving birth. When faced with someone dying during their past life regression we often ask "What was the last thing that you were thinking as you died?" We've learned that whatever that last thought was, might influence events in this lifetime.

Her thoughts were of devastation. She said "I'll never be able to see this person again; this is my one true love. I'll never be able to find this kind of love again." And in this lifetime, this was an issue she struggled with a lot, never finding perfect love. And then she found herself coming into connection with him again and finding "perfect love," and the ensuing encounter brought back all the trauma she had gone through in that previous lifetime. Together we did some clearing of that trauma, now she can see clearly who he is today is not who he was in that lifetime. Coming to know this fact helped her move on.

MEMORIES OF THE HOLOCAUST

Have you ever had a past life regression?
I'm 50 years old, so going all the way back to when I was aged 2, I still had memories of a past life. Back in those days, past lives were not something ever talked about, but at age 2, when my parents would have people over for parties for dinner, I'd run into the bedroom and hide. And my mom would come into my room and ask why I was doing that, and I would say emphatically "If I don't, someone is going to come in and take me away!" As I got older, I would beg my parents to take me to the synagogue. Interesting enough, I grew up an area where there weren't any synagogues, and there was no way of me knowing what a synagogue was, since we weren't Jewish. And my parents were at their wits end and didn't know what to do with me.

Then, probably the most terrifying experience I remember was at the age of 5. I went to take swimming classes at an old YMCA nearby, and I was in the locker room changing, and I looked up -- all the tiles were cracked and crumbling and there were these old fashioned kind of shower heads, and I took one look at the shower heads, and a teacher blew a whistle out by the pool and something in me just exploded. I got lightheaded and screamed. I started scratching and clawing and begging my mother to get me out of there.

And for many years after that, I had terrifying nightmares of sitting on a wooden step, holding on for dear life, knowing that at any moment I would be dying. I would lie in bed, just praying to wake up - and my parents took me to a pediatrician to figure out what was going on. He certainly didn't know and said it was discomfort and probably related to that. So it wasn't until I was in my 20's that I started to do more of my own in depth work into the spirit world and started to actually do some past life regressions, that I went back to the lifetime I had previous to this one.

And I remembered being in the Holocaust and the details came pretty significantly. I remembered my entire family, my mother and my father, my grandfather whom I called 'Papa' - they were all taken from me. And prior to being taken away, we were living in a small apartment, and my Papa was very close to me. And the SS came to take us away and I remember being taken into the camps and watched Papa being taken to another place and my father taken away from me. I can still feel that intense chill from being in the camp, the simple bunks and finding the place extremely cold (and in this lifetime, I continue to hate to be cold!)

I was about the age of five in the camp and I remember thinking that if I could find a way to get into the heart of this woman guard, touch her heart in some way, you know, break her ice, perhaps she would change. And so I went on a little expedition, took and picked some tiny white flowers and gave them to her; smiled at her, hoping she would take the flowers and it would open her heart. And she promptly threw the flowers down and stomped them into the ground, harshly. And when it was time for me, I remember going into the showers and hearing spirits of other women speaking to me. I knew we were going to die, and I remember hearing the spirits saying to "Remember," and to just "Look into the light."

And so some of my last emotions, my last thoughts were "Just do this." I put my hand over my mouth so I would take in as little gas as possible. I guess I wanted to be the last one to go, so then I could live a little longer and help save other lives. That was one of my last memories in that particular life, then going forward to floating above the scene and seeing souls flying past me and souls leaving; going on their way to their next journey.

One thing I brought into this life is that I've always felt it's my responsibility to save everyone, or to try to be one to stay and help others. Having done that past life regression, I can honestly say I came into this life traumatized. I had a quick turnaround from that life and quickly back. Also, when I work with people who've also gone through a traumatic past life memory, I can truly empathize.

One of the themes I emphasize in my work is "What did you learn from that life?" Mine was learning through emotions; it's powerful to know because of the stronger emotions of that lifetime. I feel so much freer in this life; I'm really at peace with that. My particular thought, I know this is controversial, was "How could anyone choose a life like that? What was the purpose in choosing a life like that with those people?" But I feel I did have a purpose. That no matter what happens on the planet, love is all that matters. And from one angle, the perpetrators had a harder life than others; probably more so. So that compassion that I had for them is probably higher and comes from a deeper place.

Do you remember the name of the camp, or your name?
The name of the camp was Bergen Belsen, my name was Hannah. Interestingly enough, many years after the regression, I took a journey to Bergen Belsen and as I walked in, I immediately knew where the barracks were. Even though everything had been torn down, there were pieces of concrete as I had seen them back them. I cried and cried and cried from the experience. But as I stood there, remembering, I could see that out of the barren ground, flowers were emerging from the concrete. It was truly transformative to see how little things change and yet to see how the grass continues to grow.

RECURRING CHARACTERS IN OUR LIVES

Has anyone from that lifetime shown up in this lifetime?
People I knew in that lifetime have shown up in this lifetime. None of my immediate family, but I did get to see them all while in the spiritual realm. One of them turned out to be my spirit guide. But there is another person who I recognized as one of the guards in the concentration camp. During my session, I recognized this person as someone I knew in high school who always pursued me romantically. For whatever reason, I just didn't feel comfortable going out with him (now I know why!) He was one of the reluctant guards with black boots. (I've always had a lot of nightmares about black boots) and he used to work the bridge and would talk to me. Of course, I didn't tell him my memory of him as a Nazi guard in a concentration camp.

When I turned 35, he called to wish me happy birthday and I told him about my past life regression, and how I'd seen him, but neglected to mention where it was, just that it was during World War II. He said "Oh, that must be why I've been collecting World War II memorabilia all my life." Turns out he's a collector of antiques and artifacts from across the world, and recently, a collector told him he'd found a special item. This item had come from a Catholic Church in France and was found in a closet after the War, the church needed money so they were selling it. He purchased it sight unseen.

So when I mentioned my past life regression to him, he said "Oh, I've got a gift for you." He put it in a frame and sent it in the mail. It was a charcoal drawing made in the Warsaw ghetto of a mother and a small child from the back, and was found later under a mattress. It also included one of the golden stars that had to be worn by the Jews in the Ghetto. When it came, I just sobbed, because I recognized the small girl in the picture as myself. Somehow they had returned to me in this life. And in some way what he was feeling was what I had been feeling – and he had found a way to give them back to me.

WHAT'S THE PURPOSE OF THIS WORK?

What do you think the significance of this past life work is?
I believe we are spiritual beings that live on this Earth. We're not Earthly beings who happen to be spiritual, but the other way around. So for me, this past life work, soulful work, is about that fact that at our core, we're this beautiful diamond and the mud that covers it are experiences in other lifetimes we've encountered. And we create these negative beliefs we have about ourselves, whether it's shame or self-hatred or unworthiness, and sometimes we have to go all the way back to the beginning - our past lives - to wash away the mud so we can uncover the beautiful diamond we are. Until you get to the source of it, you're going to be in conflict with nature until you find the source of the diamond within you.

NOTE: Debbie's interview is unusual for a number of reasons. She describes a technique of past life regression that helped a toddler with severe behavioral problems. The parents were at the end of their rope, until she was able to help the angry young child get in touch with his past life tragedy. And once he'd revealed it, his anger issues disappeared.

Later, she recounts a woman who had an affair with a married man, and the loss of the relationship was devastating. Under hypnosis, she was able to understand why she'd chosen to find this man in this life again. And finally, her own past life regression into the Holocaust mirrored the experience of "Noreen" previously mentioned. She went through difficult spiritual progression in that life that has helped formulate her current one, helping other souls.

Unaware of Michael Newton's work prior to our interview, she confirmed many of the tenets of his research. Because she wasn't aware of his work, she didn't have the benefit of having a life between life session where she might have been able to examine why she chose this difficult life that ended in the Holocaust.

In the book "Memories of the Afterlife: Life Between Lives Stories of Personal Transformation," edited by Michael Newton, there is the striking story of a 30 year old Austrian woman. During her past life regression she remembered being a German soldier hunted by U.S. forces at the close of the war. The hypnotherapist asked her to regress to an earlier, happier time, and as a male soldier, she remembers being engaged to a young Jewish girl.

The engagement subsequently fell apart in light of the politics of the era and the soldier then remembered being on the Swiss border where he was assigned to hunt down refugees trying to escape. There he encountered a truckload of refugees, and as they emerged from the truck, discovered his fiancée. "What did you do?" asked the therapist. "I shot her and the rest of them," he/she said. The soldier then remembered being violently ill afterwards, as if his body was rejecting what was happening around him.

The next session was this woman's life between life session, and in it she found herself returning to the life between lives and her soul group. It's there that out of the mist appeared the woman who had been his fiancée. He said that he was "Humiliated and horrified" to see her again, but she took his hands and said, "Don't you remember? We agreed to experience those events in this lifetime."

She reminded him of their agreement to explore the victim and perpetrator roles that had permeated that part of the twentieth century. Then the client recognized this woman in her present life, someone who'd solicited her friendship at work. In the follow up interview, she reported they'd begun working together on important environmental projects, and was grateful for being able to see their previous life together.

This is a common occurrence, as seen in "Aquaphobia," where specifically a loved one agrees to play the role of a bad person in this life so they can help the other learn lessons of a spiritual nature. This concept appears to turn traditional psychotherapy on its head, where the individual is responsible for actions because those actions may have come from childhood trauma or other psychological issues. Hard to get one's mind around this concept that people who commit crimes may not be guilty of those crimes because they were asked to do it before coming to the planet. (However, they also agreed to bear the responsibility of their actions in order to help their loved one learn a powerful truth.) But the concept of guilt and intent enter an entirely new paradigm.

It's become common practice to give prisoners the "psychopath test" as designed by Canadian criminologist Robert Hare, who studied the nature of psychopaths and discovered they respond to a set of questions and videos in the same, non-caring, non-emotional manner. (Despite not wanting to allow the justice system to use his tests, they're now offered free online.) Depending how a prisoner responds, they're categorized by the justice system on a scale of "curable" or "incurable" due to what is perceived as a genetic predisposition to being a psychopath. One might hope that the criminal justice system will begin to include, as they've done in The Netherlands, psychological evaluation of hard core criminals that may include past life regression, life between life sessions, or getting to the core of why they behave the way they do. Either way, the people who come away from these sessions reportedly find the answers to the reason they're on the planet and the apotheosis alters their behavior permanently.

But these memories of the Holocaust dove-tailed with another unusual session I was able to witness where the subject was able to ask the question "Why would anyone choose a past life with such pain?"

"As far back as I can remember I have unconsciously referred to the experiences of a previous state of existence."

- Henry David Thoreau

CHAPTER 10
THE SOUL RIVER

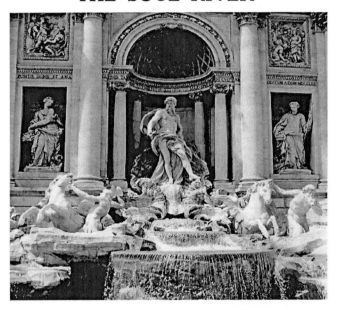

"Explore the River of the Soul; whence or in what order you have come..."

- Zoroaster

Steven is a successful television producer and an avowed skeptic when it comes to tales from the Afterlife. That being said, he has had a few psychic experiences in his life - after his mother passed away, a number of times she seemed to speak to him. In one vision, she told him talking to people in the afterlife was "the same way it works when you pick up a cell phone and try to reach someone across the planet. They pick up the phone and you have a connection." It is unusual that we can now pick up a handset and push buttons and speak to people from a mountain in Tibet, for example (as I have done); the mechanism is completely hidden, but quite logical. Could connecting to energy patterns of the dearly departed one day be as accessible to us?

Scott de Tamble is a TNI trained hypnotherapist who works in Southern California. A long haired rocker with piercing eyes and a laid back manner, Scott is one of the most talented hypnotherapists I've seen work. I arranged for him to do a session with Steven that I would film. Scott spoke to Steven prior to the session, encouraging him to bring a list of questions he might want answered in his session. After a few minutes of relaxing Steven, Scott began to take him back in time.

Steven and *Scott*

Scott: Getting younger and younger, we're in front of your home at age 12 now. Let's find a toy of Steven's at age 12.
There's a wooden toy called "Shoot the Moon." It's made of wood and it has two metal rods and a big ball bearing. The ball moves toward you and you close the rods to speed it all the way to the top. I'm good at it.

Let's move back to the stairway, getting younger, back to the womb. Be there now.
I can hear muffled voices. It feels like I have grown. There's a lot of fluid around me.

Tune into your mom's heartbeat. What's she feeling?
She's happy, but worried. She's tired of being pregnant. She wants it to be done. "Let's do this" is the feeling. I'm ready.

What's your impression of the brain you now occupy?
"Wow." (Chuckles) Just wow. I've got a smart brain.

How's the integration of soul and body?
A lot of pulsating energy. Smooth, but like stepping on a gas pedal all the way.

How does this body compare with others you may have occupied in the past?
This feels a lot faster.

Anything else about this time with your mom?
Feels very warm and safe. I can feel her love. It's very 'gracious;' it's a weird word, but it's very gracious. It's like a gift.

All right, let's float up and away from this body, out into your super conscious, expanding like circles in a pond...
NOTE: "Steven" had never been under hypnosis before, and had never had a past life regression. The session was conducted in his home, with a camera present. Prior to the session he expressed some skepticism that the process would work at all, that he might remember anything, let alone take the journey he was about to embark on.

RETURNING TO A LIFE DURING WORLD WAR II

Where are you?
Daytime. I'm outside. Standing on the street.

What kind of shoes are you wearing?
It's a dark shoe. I think I'm alone.

A big city or small town?
It's a little bit bigger, not a tiny town, but a decent sized town. I'm a girl. I'm 9 or 10.

What are you wearing?
Looks like a dress... with a bib. The whole thing is blue. Like baby blue. White kerchief or a piece of fabric. My hair is light... Blond. Very pale and fair. My eyes are blue.

Move into and behind those eyes and look out through those eyes, connecting with the thoughts and feelings of this girl. What's her name?
Either Hilda or Helga. I feel disoriented, I feel a little scared. Like I don't know where I am. I'm lost, looking for someone. My mother.

See your mother in Helga's mind's eye - what does she look like?
She's a very stern looking woman. She's wearing a scarf around her head. And a tan wool coat.

Anyone else with her?
No, by herself. She's nervous. Like we shouldn't be out here. Like a sense of like, a curfew or something. Like we need to get home.

I know you're a little scared, so let's stop the action and go back in time and tell me about your home, the place where you sleep.
It's in a small apartment in the city. I have a bed and a bedroom. A small room.

Let's go to a time you're having a meal. Who's there?
My father and my mother. We're eating dinner, but nobody's talking. Like there's something's wrong out in the world.

How about your father, what's he like?
He's about 5 foot 8. He's mostly bald.

As you're having a meal, what sort of foods are you having?
Potato. Bread. And some big bone with a little bit of meat.

Ok, let that fade away. Do you have any special interests in how you spend your time as a girl?
I like to watch what everybody's doing. I keep getting this sense that there are soldiers walking around in the street.

Is this why people are quiet?
Yeah, it's like World War II or something. Everybody's scared.

What's your family name?
The name just came in: "Lindquist."[43]

Do you know the name of the town or city?
Sounds like Svenborg, Denmark.
    NOTE: There is a Svenborg in southern Denmark, close to Germany. About 400 Jews escaped to Svenborg after Kristallnacht. The Nazis invaded April 9th, 1940, and began deporting Jews in 1943. Due to an effort by Denmark to protect Jews, only 202 were caught. With all of the session that I witnessed, I did as much forensic research as I could with names and dates. I've been told that to get the most accurate information, a client might undergo a number of sessions to get the finer points of locations and names. However, in this case, I was able to track most of what Steven remembered.

Let's go to a happy, proud moment in this life.
I'm walking for the first time. And my parents are very happy, they're clapping. I feel very happy and proud; I've done something good. (Smiles and laughs).

Let's go to a major turning point in your life.
(After a pause) I have this feeling this is a very short life. There doesn't seem to be a whole lot beyond the age of ten.

Let's move back to the moment where you were feeling a little lost. How old are you?
I'm nine. It's 1943.

Did you find your mother?
Yes, my mother finds me, and she's very nervous and rushes to get home. We shouldn't be out. We're rushing to get home.

---

[43] Later Steven said he felt he was hiding his real last name.

Let's go to the last day of Helga's life. What's happening? Where are you?
I'm outside. I'm ten years old. I'm standing.

Rise above the scene so you can observe. What happens to cause your life to end?
(After a long pause) Feels like I'm in a camp, a concentration camp.

How long have you been here?
Not very long. Nine weeks or months... They've moved us from where we were before.

Are you still with your mother or father?
No.

Let's move forward to the moment after death. You can rise from your body.
I'm floating above it.

What happened? How did you die?
I was shot.

How are you feeling about that life now?
It's kind of sad. So brief, so short.

Do you know the name of this place, this camp?
Dachau.

Before we leave, is there anything you need to do before you go?
There are just so many bodies. There are a lot of bodies.

A very unhappy scene.
Yes.

If you're ready to go then, as you move away from your body, on your journey back home, please describe what's happening. Have you started to move?
Very hard to move.

As you float there, let's relax for a moment, and know that you're now entering a soul state... (Etc.) as we enter the peaceful realm... you will receive divine help releasing any and all negative energy... We're going to meet with your friends and your teachers... Have you started to move yet?
NOTE: There are 8 records of Dachau executions of people from Svenborg or Swendborg, Denmark, according to www.jewishgen.org – having been to Dachau when I was in college, I was struck by the way Steven pronounced "Dachau" with a hard ch – the way that it's pronounced in Germany. Afterwards I asked him if he'd ever been to the location or knew anyone who died there; he did not.

ENTERING THE LIFE BETWEEN LIVES WITH A SPIRIT GUIDE

Mm-hmm. I feel like I'm being pulled away. Off to the right.

Tell me about your environment as you're being pulled away.
It's like I'm flying over the city. It's a place with white pillars or something... I can see a very blue sky up against the white pillars and there's a... not sure if it's a person, but...

A male or female?
Male.

Let's move to that person.
There's a name, a strange name. Sounds like... Luung-da.

Let's greet Long-da. Connect with him, what's the first thing you hear?
Like, "Welcome, welcome back..."

Does he have a body? What's he wearing?
It's kind of like a face, but kind of like, just light. There's a big long robe or something underneath. It's white.

If you could look through the robe and see his energy color what would that be?
It's sort of white, and yellow and a little bit pink.

I want to speak to Long-da... As I speak directly to him, he can answer my questions in your mind and you can speak his words, almost as if you're channeling his answer.
I'm trying to pronounce his name it's like... Lonnng-da. Not like English. It's a different sound.

I hope he'll forgive me if I mangle his name in my English pronunciation, so, how do you feel about this soul's performance in this lifetime? How did Helga do? It was a short life.
NOTE: As with all sessions I witnessed, when the person begins to speak as their spirit guide, their manner of speech takes on a different cadence, tone and delivery, as if channeling someone else. Certainly this manner of speaking could be invented by the person under hypnosis, but the syntax and content changes dramatically – sentence structure is different, and it's as if the person under hypnosis either struggles speaking in English, or has an ability to download bursts of information at a heightened rate. In Steven's case, the cadence and syntax reminded me of conversations I've had with Tibetan monks.

INTERVIEW WITH HIS SPIRIT GUIDE

(Steven's tone changes, his voice deeper.) Hmm. Too short.

What was the purpose of that short lifetime?
He just says "Too short." It's like it was too short to learn anything.

How was Helga's life related to Steven? What's the connection?
The connection is "Life can be short, so appreciate life." Appreciate the time you have. It's funny... I can hear myself speaking the way he talks... It's hard to speak in English. (Shakes his head)

I'm going to touch you on the forehead and it's going to sort this out in your mind, so you'll be able to speak fluently in English. What advice does your guide have for you in this current life of yours?
Life is a great gift. It's very important to love life - it's a wonderful gift.

Let's get a name for this soul of Steven and Helga; what name shall we call this soul?
Ran. Ran-dol.

So Long-da, do you feel Randol needs cleansing? Is there somewhere else you'd like to take him?
He's been many places. He's a warrior, has great spirit. Great joy.

What else?
He's a bringer of light. Helga was dark. Her whole life was just dark.

So why did Randol choose Helga, this short dark life?
Just to see and experience that... the darkness.

What's the value in seeing the darkness for a soul like Randol?
With so much light, you forget the dark. You have to be reminded every once in a while.

And why is it valuable to remember the darkness?
When you forget the darkness, you don't know it any longer. You don't know how it is for others to experience it. He needed to understand and know the dark.

Any advice how he can bring more light as Steven?
Try to forget the darkness. It's funny; I'm saying you shouldn't forget the darkness but that you should try to forget the darkness... (Laughs). But it makes sense.

Can we bring Randol somewhere to meet a group of wise beings to answer questions?
It's a like a place among the trees. Very thin trees. It's outside. Like a clearing in the woods.

NOTE: Everyone has a different experience of the location of their Council. In my case it was a room filled with light, in other cases it could be a small room, and in this instance, what appears to be a clearing outside among trees.

THE COUNCIL OF ELDERS

Let's move into that sacred space. How many beings are awaiting us?
Five. The tallest one is in the middle, it goes short then tallest then taller than short... They look almost like a crown.

How do they appear as individuals?
He's very tall, very thin. Almost like... like one of the trees, but not one of the trees.

Is the tall one the spokesman? Or are they all equal?
He's the leader, but there's a female to his left and she wants to speak too. Everyone else is quiet.

What would the female like to say?
"Welcome home. The journey is far from over. You're doing so well. We miss you, but you must continue on."

What was the life purpose as Helga?
There wasn't enough time to bring enough light, but enough to bring some good.

What is the life purpose now as Steven?
To bring much more light.

So I will speak directly to Longda and he can speak through your mind "Was my experience of being a gunslinger true?[44]"
You thought you were the gunslinger, but you were not. You were the good one; it was the bad one who shot you.

What was Randol's name in that lifetime?
Jed Ellis.

And where was that?
Tomb... Tombstone, Arizona. 1869.[45]

Where was he born in that lifetime?
Sedalia. Kansas? Or Arkansas. [46]

---

[44] While having a deep tissue massage, Steven spontaneously remembered a past life as a gunslinger who shot a man in the street.
[45] According to the web, there was man named Ellis shot in the Dodge House bar in Tombstone in July 1873.
[46] There's a Sedalia in both.

Let's show him something about that lifetime.
Wearing a bowler. Pinstripe suit. I'm a watchmaker.

Let's go to the scene where you get shot... Why does the gunslinger shoot you?
He's angry. He's somehow picked on me. I knew about him. I wanted to stay away. I was visiting, got involved with the wrong guy. I didn't know he was so bad...

Is there any lesson in that past life?
Better watch out who you're talking to. Sometimes you say the wrong thing to the wrong person.

And his life as Helga? Randol chose that as well?
Yes. "But when you gotta go, you gotta go."

Are you a teacher?
I am. My children (in this life) are in my class. I'm teaching them to be bringers of light.

Why has Steven felt he's had success ripped away under strange circumstances?
It would be too easy the other way. It's like a game of hide and seek when you're not really hiding - it would be easy to find you... it's just a game.

NOTE: It was unusual for Steven to mention a town he'd never heard of, but that exists (as he said) in both Arkansas and Kansas, and the name of a victim, Ellis, that is verifiable in the rolls of people who were shot in the infamous Tombstone.

THE POINT OF LIVING A DIFFICULT LIFE

What's the point in having it taken away?
Otherwise there's no game. (Laughs). It's too easy the other way.

Is this something he agrees to? That he does himself?
I don't do it myself, it's been arranged though. It was a bad choice to arrange it. But otherwise there would be no challenge.

Let me ask your female elder on your council what's the purpose of having challenges like this?
It's about patience and understanding, it's to learn about trust and patience.

Why did Steven purchase a home in Montana?
The watchmaker had a place like his (Steven's) home in Montana… It's grassland. Big land. There's lots of space – it's big enough to fill it.

NOTE: Steven told me that at some point in his life he was drawn to buying a ranch in the mountains. Having grown up in the suburbs of Chicago, it's not something he could put his mind around why he wanted to own a ranch, but he'd done so, and spent many weekends there raising various farm animals.

Why does he recently have a fear of heights?
It's from falling. Not in this lifetime. He was climbing rocks, big rocks. He died at the age of 36-40. It was in the southwest United States. 1821. He was a Navajo Indian brave.

Why has this fear of heights come into his life? Why has he become aware of this fear?
Nothing is forever. You can't reach the sky when you're a human being. Life comes and goes.

I'm addressing the elders now. (Reading from Steven's list of questions) He wants to know if he's known his wife in a previous lifetime.
Yes. When I was the Navajo I was married to her, a Navajo also. Long black hair. She's a difficult woman. (Smiles). She's strong willed.

What's her name?
Tee too ha. It means "bird in flight."[47]

What's your name?
Hay koo ma.[48] It means "long lizard." He was a Fearless man.

What was the connection between that past life and this life?
Be crazy fearless. Fear nothing; be bold.

What about his competitive streak? Why does he hate losing?
It comes from being human... That's part of the human being. Because where we come from (in the life between lives), there's no winning or losing.

Being here, we enjoy this.
This is the game, yeah.

Is there a pattern to the lives he's lived? What is it and why?
The pattern is always to bring that special something... It's the light - the promise is the light, the bringing of the light. This is his pattern, over and over.

NOTE: In many between life sessions, people describe an intense light that permeates the Universe – some ascribe it qualities of healing and love or compassion. This light is apparently contained in everything, and by channeling it in a positive manner it can be used to heal or help people.

---

[47] "Thi'thuNwan (TEE-too-wah) is a Dakota word for "Prairie dweller." Te-wa is a Hopi word from the Navajo region.

[48] The "how-ku-ma" tribe were in the Western United States in the 1800's.

BRINGING THE LIGHT FROM HEAVEN INTO THIS LIFE

Bring the light? Can you put that in other terms?
It's to bring what is there in this other place (between lives) - to bring to this place. To bring peace and the knowing that all is well.

About the specific purpose of this lifetime as Steven, what's the main life purpose?
To bring light to many people.

Through his work in the media?
This is his tool. We've never had this before, to be able to reach so many people.

Does he have specific lessons in this lifetime?
The life of Helga was very shocking, very upsetting; it's like "Let it go, shake it away."

He's still having residue?
It's the source of his doubt. The world can be shocking, horrible and bad. Her life was to show him how bad it could be.

A TRIP TO THE SOUL RIVER

Let's halt this and take him to a place to cleanse him of this darkness and doubt.
The soul river.

Let's go there. Tell me about this place.
This is where one washes the soul.

You all walk in together?
Yes. With the elders. This is... These are the waters to forget. The waters to wash clean.

Let the water cleanse you. Be there with the elders. Stay as long as you need to.
(Lips moving) I'm aware... That (my life as Helga) it burned my soul. That time burned my soul. (He takes a deep breath...)

Let the waters soothe your soul. Rest now. While you're resting, etch this in your mind. Your body and soul can always remember this place. You can return to this place of healing anytime you wish. Take your time; tell me when you're ready.
I can go now.

Did you wash away the trauma? How do you feel?
I've carried that a long time. It's better now.

What's the message you got from that time?
I never knew the darkness could be *so*... It was really dark.

Now you have a taste of that, and you can help others who've experienced dark times.
Now there's no need for doubt.

Let's move back to the clearing and ask the elders, perhaps the tall one, to speak for us and tell us what it is he needs to know now as Steven.
Bring the Navajo warrior to your spirit here. Be not afraid, don't doubt, just bring it all.

Why has Steven been brought to this session? What does he need to get from this experience?
This was all part of the plan that you created. This is, this was what you set out to do. No one wrote this for you. You wrote it for yourself.

So why at this moment in his life is he having this experience?
You have enough time to do it. Play in it. There's plenty of time.

Steven, is there anything you would like to ask the council? Take your time.
Give me your strength, give me your knowledge. Be my courage.

How do they respond?
"We are here for you. Yes, of course."

Let me ask what he needs to touch that strength and courage, how can he contact you to be able to have that flow through him?
"Don't doubt it; we are there for you." Be bold and fearless.

Any messages from the council for this soul here?
"All this you know." And "You make us laugh." (Chuckles).

NOTE: Scott, the hypnotherapist, also found this an unusual journey, one he'd never heard before. Certainly references to the "River of Souls" can be found throughout literature, usually described as the River Styx where souls flow like a river. But in this instance, Steven refers to it as a place of healing, a cleansing place, where one can soothe the trauma from a previous lifetime, in his case, the short life and death of a young girl in Dachau, by dipping into its waters.

A MATTER OF PERSPECTIVE

If your guide Long-da is still here with us, perhaps there's something else he'd like to show you. Something amazing for you to see.
Hmm. (nods). Long-da is showing me that in all the world of light, the darkness around is only one small speck... (Holds up fingers to indicate tiny) that's the right perspective. A tiny, tiny speck, it's nothing. The darkness seemed like everything; but it's nothing.

What is he telling you by showing you this?
(Laughs). "Don't believe in nonsense."

Perhaps Long-da will suggest another place to visit.
Long-da says to come to the "place of knowing."

Excellent, let's do that then.
This is a place - it's a field of light. And we step into it… You step into the light, to know, but to be <u>here</u>. To be human and know.

Have you stepped in?
Yes. (Eyes moving under the lids rapidly, head going back and forth. He nods).

Tell us about your experience here.
It reminds me of when I came into this body, it's "Wow." (Laughs). The knowing.

So that's flowing into you?
Mm-hm. Electrical. This is the flow of energy, it's endless energy.

So why has Longda brought you here today, to this place of knowing?
This is where you came from. So you can know where you came from in this life.

    NOTE: This experience of feeling the endless flow of energy that permeates the Universe is described in a number of sessions in the book.

A FINAL MEETING WITH HIS PARENTS

Is there something you're still yearning for? Someone you want to say hello to?
I'd like to see my parents again.

Let's do that. Long-da can guide us. Let's go and be with them.
Yes, I'm feeling much love. I'm feeling their love.

Are you in their presence?
Both of them, but they are in a different form now. They're energy light. They're like guides.

Are you closer to one of them?
They're standing together.

This is your chance to embrace, flow into them. Say in your heart whatever you want to say.
They're saying that I was their teacher. Strange. I thought they were mine.

What did they learn from you?
They learned how to laugh. (Smiles). They learned to believe in the extraordinary.

Do they have any thoughts or messages to you for your current life?
They're giving back to me what I gave to them. They say I gave them the extraordinary and they're giving it back to me. They're reminding me of everything from where they are.

What sort of activities are they involved in now?
They're in school. They're learning to come back. They're picking up a few things before coming back. Which will be very soon.

Will they be born before you pass?
Yes, I think so.

Do you know what land they're going to be in? Any details?
(Laughs). My mother says she's going to Wisconsin.

Anything else that they wish to share with you before we leave them?
They just said "Play on."

Ok then, kind of like a group hug, your immortal self joining with your current self, Steven... You are living now as Steven... I'll count from one to ten..."
A number of profound moments happened in Steven's session. I've known him since high school, and I know him to be a funny, smart guy who has a deep philosophical streak. He's been pretty successful at every endeavor he's attempted, and continues to be a gracious person. He was profoundly moved by being able to cleanse his soul in the Soul River, and meet his parents during the process. He basically hit all the same bases that everyone does under the Newton method of hypnosis; his spirit guide, his council of Elders, his loved ones and family. I think he's not convinced he didn't make it all up, but perhaps when he sees the other interviews in this book, he'll see how uniform his experience was. At least I hope so.

He continues to be a successful television producer and frequently spends weekends at his ranch out in the country, albeit with a clearer connection to his lives as a watchmaker and a fierce Navajo warrior.

One of the usual criticisms of reincarnation is that "Everyone remembers being someone famous, like Cleopatra." Perhaps this was common in mental hospitals in the 1960's, but most therapists that are trying to help patients overcome a past life memory won't dwell long in a previous incarnation, famous of otherwise. However, with the ease the Internet gives us to do forensic research into past life stories, it's just a matter of time before someone finds Elvis.

"With all your science can you tell me how it is, and whence it is, that light comes into the soul?"

- Henry David Thoreau

Chapter 11
ELVIS' GUITAR PLAYER
& CAROLE LOMBARD

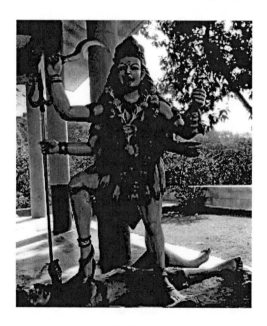

"I have been born more times than anybody except Krishna."

- Mark Twain

Inevitably the subject of reincarnation swings around to famous people. Over the years, numerous people have come forth to claim they were reincarnates of celebrities. Sometimes people who claim to be someone famous in their past life have something to gain or benefit from the revelation, and due to the abundance of information now available through the internet, it's fairly easy to create a memory of a past life -- if one had the time, inclination and motivation, that is.

One thing Jimmy Quast mentioned in his interview; "In the afterlife, there is no hierarchy, no one gets to horde the jelly beans." We're all on equal footing in the afterlife, according to these people, some of us may be older souls than others, but we may still go through a number of lifetimes to examine a particular flaw in our overall makeup we want to address. I've had two examples of celebrity pop up in my interviews, and I considered them interesting anecdotes. The question isn't "Why were you famous in a previous lifetime and you're not now?" but "Why did you choose that previous lifetime and why did you choose this one, and what's the common theme between the two?"

Colleen-Joy Page is a tall, blue eyed brunette from Johannesburg,[49] a motivational speaker, life coach and author who teaches online courses via her website.

INTERVIEW WITH COLLEEN-JOY PAGE

How did you come to this work?
Colleen-Joy Page: At the age of four and a half, I had a near death experience during surgery to remove a large tumor from behind my right eye and I began asking those big questions like "Who am I?" and "Why am I here?" from a very young age. I was haunted by an image of a tunnel of light, I felt homesick for the first 26 years of my life, and I had many flashbacks, many past life memories. I struggled to reconcile my inner experiences with what the world was telling me was true, so I went on a bit of a quest to find my own truth.

When I came across Newton's first book, "Journey of Souls," I found myself crying with joy because when you have your own inner experiences, you're always left with a slight feeling of being uncertain whether to trust them. There's no one to confirm them, or validate them, and here I was reading words from someone who lived half a planet away from me, who'd spent thirty years of his life researching these accounts of people remembering themselves as souls, remembering their other lives and more importantly remembering what it was to be a soul between lifetimes. These were exactly the experiences I'd remembered throughout my life - to read the words was just so moving and incredible.

Many years later he came to South Africa and a friend of mine arranged that visit. I attended some seminars and realized here was a way to gift the world with a method to finding out who they really were.

---

[49] http://www.colleen-joy.com/

SOUL MEMORIES

Tell us about what's the experience of a life between lives? A typical journey?
A typical "life between life" regression is about four and a half hours long; one needs a certain level of trance depth in order to access the mind that has the soul memories. One of the things Michael's work has demonstrated is that the physical body has a mind of its own - a kind of physical ego and that this physical ego is quite different to the soul's ego.

The challenge for the LBL therapist is to attain enough trance-depth to bypass the conscious mind and its ability to interfere with the super conscious mind. You have your soul's memories or wisdom trying to come through, and the human mind is like a bouncer preventing those deep wisdoms from emerging. The LBL process is the best possible route to getting a person past their physical conscious mind and into the super conscious mind where these memories are stored.

Typically it starts with an induction, a deepening of trance, then current life regression to warm the person's mind up. From the current life, we go back to the womb where the person is able to recount the experience of being a fetus, and then from the womb we move back to a past life memory specifically looking for the death scene, because we've found through the death scene memory, a person's mind is more easily able to open to their soul memories.

After the person passes through the death scene, they start to remember what it is to be a soul and then there is a sequence of events quite similar for most people, although they can be in different order. They are met by a loving soul mate, a friend in spirit, or their teacher or their guide in spirit. And from then on there is an orientation as well as a de-briefing of the life they've just lived, and then the soul moves into the normal activities of the spirit world.

Sometimes this might involve some kind of celebration, where they are reunited with their spiritual friends and family, sometimes there's a bit of rest. Very often the soul carrying the baggage of a human experience needs some kind of healing on the other side, to fully acclimatize to its soul consciousness, and so there is usually healing or restoration. At some point, the soul is taken before its council or wise elders or teachers, where in a very loving, caring and supportive way, the soul is given the opportunity to reflect on the life just lived and on the bigger picture of their many existences, their many lifetimes. They review the lessons and themes that are part of their own spiritual journey and their own spiritual involvement.

CHOOSING OUR NEXT LIFE

How do we choose our next incarnation?
One of the things that surprises people the most about their own memories of being a soul is just how much free will there is. Every soul chooses its own lifetime. It's a very careful choice, usually a very sacred choice, but each soul is given more

than one choice. The soul looks over potential lifetimes on Earth and is also able to scan potential future timelines. We have realized through the life between life work there is never one set path, you don't incarnate with a set beginning and a set ending mind - there's no *one future timeline*, in fact time seems to be more like a tree with many branches. It's up to us as souls to navigate those branches to the best of our ability and to make our choices and live with those choices. So life selection is taken very seriously.

We often choose based on what we desire to learn in an incarnation; every now and then a soul will choose a lifetime for rest and recreation, but usually we choose a body for what that body will give to us in terms of learning. Also, there's often a theme of service where the soul might choose a lifetime to serve humanity in some way, or to improve on their skills. If a soul is very interested in healing, it may choose a lifetime with a broken body, or with an illness in mind, in order to enhance its own healing skills and knowledge.

Always wisdom is uppermost in mind. We choose to incarnate to harvest wisdom from the lifetime, to gain direct experience and knowledge so that we are improved as beings, so that we are expanded as beings, so that we have more wisdom, understanding and compassion.

Souls choose a lifetime very carefully; they have meetings with the other souls they're going to incarnate with, they have meetings and preparation with their guides where they review all the possibilities ahead of them. And the real intention is to make the most of every lifetime because lifetimes are treated as very precious, sacred experiences.

THE JOURNEY FROM THE AFTERLIFE BACK TO LIFE

And once they choose the life they're going to come into, how does that process unfold?
One of the most exciting things an LBL therapist can be witness to is the merger of the soul into human form, because you have two minds at play; the mind and consciousness of the body and the consciousness of the soul. This delicate merger of these two quite contrasting consciousnesses is just an unbelievable thing to listen to and to experience.

When you ask questions that relate to the body, it's as if the person speaks very much from the body perspective; the confining feeling of the womb perhaps, or the nurturing feeling coming from the mother, or even the distress of being in the womb, that's a very personal experience. But the moment you ask a question that relates more to the soul, there's a switch to a more peaceful, slightly detached and yet very loving perspective from the soul. You hear incredible descriptions of how the soul takes its energy and works very skillfully with the human brain and the human body to make the merger a good one.

Each soul has its own preferences when it merges with the human fetus, some at three to four months, and others wait until the last moment to get in and work with the human form. But there has to be a melding of energies, of minds, and it can take the first few years to have that merger fully complete.

Most souls still feel that slight detachment for the first few years, where they'll even go away from the baby body sometimes when it's sleeping, to come back to comfort it. Some accounts of children's invisible friends are children feeling or experiencing their own souls with them, until the soul becomes entrenched in the body for the duration of that lifetime.

GOLDEN APPLES

And have you had your own personal regression?
It was of being a woman in Copenhagen. I had flashes of having a young daughter, of plating or braiding her hair, and then a flash of a well, then suddenly overwhelmed with incredible sadness and grief as I remembered my daughter had fallen down a well, and what struck me was that despite a lack of clear visual information, the emotion was so absolutely raw.

I remembered dying by a fountain in Copenhagen; I remembered leaving my energy in the fountain as a way to gift to this fountain in the middle of Copenhagen. I did a little research on the internet and managed to find this fountain is one of the oldest landmarks in Copenhagen. [50] The image of an apple tree has always been a very personal thing for me; I use apples and apple trees as symbols in my teaching work. I discovered the name is "The fountain of golden apples" and shortly after my death in that life, they remodeled it and put apples atop the spouts, a lovely little personal affirmation of my past life memory.

You mentioned something about past life memories of your two daughters?
My eldest daughter used to have a lot of nightmares; at the age of 3 ½ I was walking past her bedroom, and heard her moaning and grinding her teeth. She was speaking as well, so I just crept in and heard her shouting "Run, run, the Huns are coming!" then "Help, I'm slipping on the ice!" Of course in South Africa, it rarely snows, so my children have never had the experience of being on ice, the next morning I asked her "Do you know who the Huns are, sweetheart?" She looked at me and said "No, mummy." So she had no conscious memory of that.

Once I was hanging up the washing and that same daughter looked at me and said, "Mummy, once I was on a ship and I tripped and I fell off the ship." Little moments like that sort of crop up every now and then. My younger daughter was listening to a new release of an Elvis Presley song that came out a couple of years back, "A little less talk, a little less action.[51]" It was a mix of a modern singer plus the original Elvis song, and she was singing along with the words. Her dad asked

---

[50] The fountain re-opened 26 May 1892, on occasions, golden apples bounce on the water jets of the fountain." Wikipedia.

[51] The Remix of a "Little Less Conversation" was featured in the film "Ocean's 11" in 2001

"How do you know the words to this song?" She said "Well, I used to be in the band with the man who was singing." Of course we were all a bit skeptical. Then she said "I played the guitar with him and I had an accident and I hurt my hand, and I couldn't play anymore.[52]" So when they say "in another life" or "Mommy, I was this…" I think it's time to start paying attention."

Certainly it's possible to find out the number of guitarists who played with Elvis who've passed away before the time her daughter was born. According to Carol Bowman, a child's past life memory doesn't change from day to day the way a fantasy does. Or a child may filter it from their present frame of reference, even when remembering events in a previous life. It's like remembering a film you saw before you could speak – not all the imagery might make sense.

I interviewed Chuck Frank,[53] a hypnotherapist who lives and works in Hollywood, Florida; he had an interesting tale to tell about his cat, Al. Chuck's got an incredible presence about him, his energy and sense of humor jump through the phone.

INTERVIEW WITH CHUCK FRANK

RM: What drew you to this work in the first place?
CF: It seems I've been groomed for this my entire life. I was born into a family that made monuments and mausoleums for cemeteries for 3 generations, and worked in the family business until I was 45 years old. I realized there was a pattern customers had; the shock of losing a loved one threw their system out of harmony and every week I would hear the same tragic stories.

I had a copy of "Life After Life"[54] on my desk and I'd casually introduce the research of a doctor whose patients had near death experiences to our clients. The experiences were similar: they saw a light went towards it and the light had a consciousness to it where they felt love and peace, and so on. This immediately changed the level of energy in the discussion; there was now a ray of hope for something to have happened to their beloved that was positive.

In 1973 I met a spiritual teacher who showed me a technique to see and feel the Spiritual Light within myself and I've been meditating on this Light for over 37 years now. I realized I have an ability to help souls cross over from the physical body to the loving, peaceful spirit realm, not in the Jack Kevorkian way, but with loving guidance that helps a soul connect to their spiritual helpers in the non-physical realm.

---

[52] There are a number of guitarists who left Elvis and the band over the years, but I've yet to find one who "hurt his hand." Perhaps some reader might be able to shed light on this one.

[53] hypnosisarts.com

[54] "Life After Life" by Dr. Raymond Moody (1975)

D-DAY IN WORLD WAR II

What was your first past life regression like?
I found myself in World War II landing on one of the beaches during the invasion of France where I got shot in the chest and was dying on the beach. There were the most intense scenes, with planes and bombs and thousands of people shooting and bleeding and dying and crying and screaming. And there were people coming to help me and I was telling them it was OK, and not to worry about me. I enjoyed watching all the action, which was amazing.

I was able to leave and come back to my body at will and I was accompanied by this beautiful light being. There were all these souls around me dying, and were having the hardest time transitioning from the body into the spirit realm; they were in total agony. Here I was able to move effortlessly into the spirit realm and these other fellows were screaming from the depths of their souls in fear.

I'd already left my body, so I went to this fellow wrapped my arms around him, comforted him and helped him up and into the light and helped him connect again with his spiritual guide. I kept doing this again and again. It dawned on me this was the reason for my existence on Earth; when all hell had broken loose, I was needed to help souls transition. It was a profound and amazing realization.

A TYPICAL LBL SESSION

What's the typical LBL session like for your clients?
I've done around 70 LBL sessions, and it's one of the highlights of my life to see a person walk in the door, be shy and nervous because they don't know if they can do the session, then 5 or 6 hours later when the session is over, they walk out the door a changed person. They have a knowing confidence, a sense of not only relief, but a sense of mastery and a deep understanding of their life, their purpose, and how all the details and experiences fit together like a puzzle; for me this is priceless. It's priceless to watch a human being change before my eyes in just a few short hours.

A CAT AND A GRANDFATHER

Have you had any unusual sessions before?
I had a cat named Al. He was crying really loud when he caught my attention in a store; I went over to see why this little guy was making all that noise, our eyes met and I felt like he was the most beautiful cat I'd ever seen, even though I'd never been friendly with any cat. I took him home.

The first night he jumped onto the bed and crawled into my armpit and slept there the entire night; he spent roughly the next 20 years in the same position. Needless to say we became best friends. Recently, when he was too old and weak to stand up I had the vet come and put him to sleep. The entire time Al kept his eyes glued to mine; we both knew these were our last moments together. About a half hour after the vet left, I sat down to meditate.

I wondered if my little friend had adjusted to the spirit realm. I decided if I could help humans go into the spirit realm, why couldn't I do the same with Al? I saw him in my mind's eye as a ball of energy, and proceeded to imagine opening my heart and picturing a golden white light streaming from the center of my heart into his heart, the two beams of light connecting. I learned this "Heart melding" technique from a vet actually, Dr. Ryan of Assisi Animal Hospital, she taught the technique in an "animal communication" workshop. I use this technique for my clients; they tell me it's their favorite part of the session.

During the session I realized part of Al's calling in this life was to help me develop the unconditional love I'd learned from him over the past 20 years. This was really heartwarming for me to experience and at that moment I felt his soul fully adjusted to the spirit realm. It felt great.

Have you had any other unusual LBL sessions without a patient being present?
One day about 10 years ago my friend and I were meeting someone in a metaphysical bookstore, in Jupiter, Florida. A man who worked there, who said he was a psychic, called out to me as I was leaving the store, "Chuck, I've got a message for you from someone on the other side." I asked who it was. He told me my grandfather wanted to apologize to me. I asked which grandfather and he told me "On your father's side." I said, "Screw him, he was a pain in the ass when he was alive, why would I want to talk to him now?" My friend and I laughed and walked out of the store.

Ten years later, I found that indeed, my grandfather Charlie was hovering around. During a session, I made peace with him, and then helped him move upward to meet his spirit guide, whom he called Harry. Harry encapsulated Charlie in a golden white light and took him to visit his Soul Group. It turned out everyone in his soul group appeared to be under ten years old, along with my grandfather. (I'd only known him as an old man. He was poor and known as a real tough guy.) All the kids in his soul group were happy and playful and they told Charlie he'd become a grouchy old man and reminded him how playful he was at this young age, and how good it is to be joyous.

His spirit guide then took him to his Council of Elders, I saw the entire council looking very solemn and serious. The chairperson said, "You forgot you had a choice each second, and each breath. You were out of balance. You forgot your heart." The chairperson went to Charlie, put his hand on his heart and appeared to energize him. He said "You turned against your own children and grandchildren and they avoided you. You stomped on their dreams and creativity and said things like "You're nothing but a shoemaker." That being said, we're glad you're here. So, are you ready to play again, feel joy again? Help others versus judge and criticize?"

"Yes," my grandfather answered. "We can help," said the chairperson. "You can start by hugging your grandchild. He brings people here, and we don't usually let anyone observe." I felt my grandfather come over to hug me, and then the entire council joined in for this incredible group hug. The chairperson said to me, "Your job is done." Charlie appeared realigned with the essence of the universe, love, his heart healed. I had just witnessed this most beautiful scene. I started to leave, but before I did, the lead council member smiled at me and said "By the way, your cat Al says "Hi."

INTERVIEW WITH "PATTY" AKA CAROLE LOMBARD

Chuck contacted me recently about a past life regression he did with a client in Orlando whom I'll call Patty. He said during her session she described a particular place in California she'd never heard of before; Barstow. She remembered being dressed in a red halter top and going to a party in Los Angeles; Chuck asked her if she knew anyone at the party. She said, "There's Cecil;" when he asked who it was, she said "DeMille." She told him her good friend Barbara Stanwyck was there, and while they were talking Clark Gable arrived at the party. She said she and Clark were old friends, and they left together in his long, white convertible. She said they went back to his place, which she thought was "awfully furnished" and consummated their flirtation with a bout in the bedroom. Patty told Chuck detailed things about this past life and according to Chuck "there were deep emotions attached to the details, which is for me a sign of her actually "being there.""" He says that when he asked what her name was, and she said "Carole." And asking her last name, she said "Lombard."

She then described traveling to "somewhere in the Midwest where she was with her mother and selling War Bonds." She said she remembered "It was cold," and she was eager to get back to California. She said the plane refueled in Las Vegas, and then a few moments after takeoff, it crashed. She remembered waking up on the plane with people shouting and general panic, but wasn't awake long; the plane crashed and killed her. Chuck has only had this one session with her; they didn't get to an LBL.

I interviewed Patty over the phone and she later sent me Frank's direct notes from the session. She is a math teacher from Detroit, living in Orlando. She told me about her life in great detail; when she was a little girl, she had a "strange memory" thinking she could fly until she was about four years old. She said growing up, she felt she always knew she was going to be an actress, and went to pursue a career in New York. She met her husband there, and together with their daughter moved to Los Angeles for his work.

She said she was aware Carole Lombard was an actress, but hadn't seen any of her films, nor knew much about her life in detail while living in LA. Patty studied acting and went on auditions, but when she became pregnant a second time, she gave up trying to have a career in Hollywood, and convinced her husband to return to her native Detroit. It was there that she had her first past life regression with a Newton trained therapist, but in that incident, the life that presented itself was during the Civil War, a widow living in the South during the hard times of post war. She saw her current husband in that lifetime, and said when she looked up specific names and dates from the session they were accurate; she felt her session was a legitimate form of therapy, and was eager to try it again.

She found Chuck listed on the Newton website, and called him up for a session. She said she was surprised to find herself remembering the life of the actress, and when I spoke to her, she still hadn't taken the time to view any of Carole Lombard's films. "I'll have to get around to that and see if anything looked familiar." She said she was still trying to process the session, doesn't have any plans to benefit from it in any way, and was kind enough to allow me to tell her story for the first time.

Was she really Carole Lombard? I think it would require a number of sessions under a number of protocols to get to a clear answer, along with the help of forensic historians. Certainly the details of her story coincide with Carole's life and death; Lombard appeared with Clark Gable in a film before she married him – it was after her divorce from fellow thespian William Powell that she wound up marrying Clark Gable. They were famous for having a simple home in Encino, where she would putter around her garden, another memory that came up during Patty's session. The details of the Mayfair Ball where Lombard ran into Gable again (who *was* married at the time) were accurate as well, including the convertible that Gable owned at the time.[55] And finally, the details of her death were accurate; she was back in the Midwest selling War Bonds with her mother during the winter, and it was on her return to California, after the plane refueled in Las Vegas, that it crashed into a nearby mountain.

That being said, the actress Emma Roberts, niece of Julia, claims a psychic in Michigan told her she was the reincarnation of Carole Lombard. According to Adrian Finkelstein, MD, who wrote a book about one of his clients being the reincarnation of Marilyn Monroe, claims one of his clients was once Carole Lombard. (Lot of Lombards going around, aren't there?) I include this account not to claim that Patty was actually Carole Lombard, but to include that there are both famous and non-famous memories from patients – some dramatic, others less so. This research emphasizes not who you were, but *why* you were. What is it about this past life that you can bring forth into this life, and benefit from knowing it?

In light of this research, my question to Patty is; why did you choose that life during the Civil War, and why did you choose that life of an actress, and why did you choose the life of a math teacher? What do they have in common? And it's through these interviews that we find that energy transfer seems to be one of the

---

[55] Gable's 1935 Duesenberg matches this description, and the time as well. It's currently at the Blackhawk auto museum in Danville, Ca. His better known convertible was a 1938 black Packard.

major components of our choice of next life – as an actor, one is able to affect people's lives through getting them to experience emotions through laughter or tears, as a teacher, the energy transfer is more immediate, actually spending time with little souls every day and helping them figure out the paths of their lives. Patty said during her Civil War memory, she saw that her current husband was her husband during that lifetime as well. That they're working out issues in this life that remain from that one. The circle remains unbroken.

But if it's true that we choose our parents, then what does that say about adoption?

"Friends are all souls that we've known in other lives. We're drawn to each other. That's how I feel about friends. Even if I have only known them a day, it doesn't matter. I'm not going to wait till I have known them for two years, because anyway, we must have met somewhere before, you know."

- George Harrison

Chapter 12
OH, THERE YOU ARE

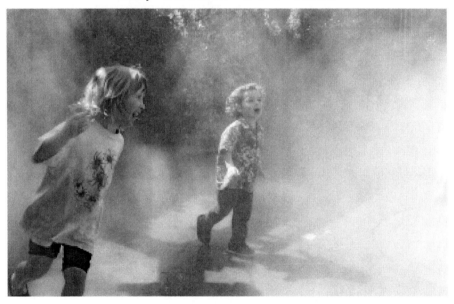

"An invisible red thread connects those who are destined to meet, regardless of time, place, or circumstance. The thread may stretch or tangle, but it will never break."

- Chinese Proverb

Sandra Bullock, the Oscar winning actress, recounted the first day she met her adopted son, an African American baby from New Orleans; "The first time I met Louis it was like the whole outside world just got quiet. He was so small, so still. All the trivial things that I had allowed to take up so much of my time just didn't have room in life anymore. All I said when I met him was, "Oh, there you are." It was like he had always been a part of our lives."[56]

The actress Meg Ryan had a similar story about the adoption of her child; "I am convinced, completely convinced that there was nothing random about (the adoption)," she told Redbook in its May, 2007 issue. "(The baby) and I got to meet each other in this way at this time… I saw that face and *I just knew* we were related."

From an interview in a magazine about adoption; "The oddest thing happened… I am sitting in church and a feeling overwhelms me that… a series of events had already unfolded, decisions had been made that would lead to the abandonment of the girl who would become my daughter. It wasn't that the outcome had been decided, but her destiny had become fixed. We were going down two roads that would eventually converge."[57]

When my daughter was born, she came out speaking, literally. Before she emerged from the womb, she opened her eyes and looked at her startled dad and said "Heggadaba!" I spent years asking Sufis, Shamans, and Rabbis if they'd ever heard such a word. None could help. Finally, some years later, I was asking her about it, and she said "It's kind of a made up language in the afterlife. When I saw you I said it. It sort of means, "Oh, there you are!"

"Noel" is a successful Hollywood executive. He came out to Hollywood in the 1960's and went to work in a literary agency where his legendary boss represented some of the most high powered people in the film and literary world. His clients included world famous authors, many whose books have been adapted into films. I met him in the 1980's when I talked him into representing me as a writer. He and his wife recently adopted a little girl from Asia. I've taken steps to disguise who he really is, as I've done with other people who generously allowed me to film their personal life between life sessions. This interview took place in his office overlooking Beverly Hills.

Session with *Scott De Tamble and* Noel

Scott begins by deepening Noel's journey and about 40 minutes in he asks him to stop at age 12 to see what he remembers.
That year, the age of 12 was about the worst year of my life. I have very negative feelings about that year. My step father and mother were constantly fighting. Eventually they decided to separate.

---

[56] People Magazine 4-28-2010
[57] Adoptive Parents Magazine, 2002 "Was It Destiny That Matched Me With My Child? By Bonnie Perkel

Ok then, let's go back to the stairway. Let's go back to age 4... Describe some fun activity.
It'd be difficult to describe any fun. Rolling up and down the small hillside in front of my home - fun was to get out of that house. At four, my mother had just married my stepfather and I guess I was ushered into this house, my room was set up and that was that. I learned to be by myself. I had a group of imaginary animals I used to hide under my blanket before I'd go to sleep. I didn't feel any warmth or any protection or comfort in the family so I turned to my imagination.

What sort of animals?
Basically furry ones - chipmunks, baby squirrels because they were small and I could fit them under the blanket and I could cover them up so nobody would see them - I didn't want my Mother or Father to walk in the room and see I was relaxed, or feeling comforted or feeling loved.

Remember a happier moment.
The movie, *The Song of the South*, was something I remember very vividly, as the songs were being sung; I felt very happy, and took with me this *Mr. Bluebird On My Shoulder*, it made me feel good as I sang it to myself as a child. "Everything is natural, everything is satisfactual..."

Let's go back to the stairway... Moving down; four, three, two... Nine months. Before birth, and in the womb. Feel the protection of this warm environment. Do you feel comfortable?
I'm comfortable in the fetal position because I can hear noises from outside; but I want to say if I could have been aborted, they would have - I've always felt I was not someone my mother wanted.

Tune into your mother's thoughts and feelings... what are you picking up?
What I pick up is she just needed to get married. She needed to have me right away - but it was not what she wanted.

Let's be there before birth and tune into your mother's emotions. What do you sense?
She was nervous and worried, depressed. It followed me all my life, leads to my lack of self-esteem, the shyness, the sensitivity. Rolled up in that feeling of not being worthwhile enough.

This starts before you're born?
It does.

    NOTE: I've known Noel for 30 years, and these feelings of worthlessness and trauma from his youth are news to me. As the camera filmed him, I was nearby at a computer terminal, and when he recounted the following life of a soldier in France and London, I was able to track down links to this soldier by the time the session was finished.

A JOURNEY TO LONDON

Let's go ahead and move away from this time with your mother. Begin to disengage and float up and away... (Etc.) Let's move into your most recent previous lifetime, before Noel. Feel yourself moving through a tunnel... finding yourself in a significant moment in a previous lifetime... (etc) Be there now.

I'm someplace in Europe; seems like old London. It's daytime, I have on a black top hat and black suit - and I'm slinking around the London streets.

You're outside in the street.

I'm shielding something and looking for someplace to put it. A document. I'm holding it, pushing into my jacket so no one will see it. From a church, they gave it to me to deliver to somebody. I've got those pointy shoes like elves, very wide brim, and dark hair. My face - my skin is whiter, my eyes are now dark, dark brown eyes, and my nose was straight, very handsome. Medium sized man, I'm 36 years old.

What's your name?
Alfred.

Notice those eyes of Alfred's... move into and look through them... Connect with the thoughts and feelings of Alfred.

Alfred... he feels confused. They gave me a document and I don't know where to go with it. I see myself in this world looking out and I'm kind of befuddled, not sure what to do.

Let's stop the action for a moment and go back earlier in Alfred's life...

I see myself being born in a small barn like structure, taken care of by two women, they have shawls on, in their 60's - I do have a little rocking bed I sleep in... one is rocking me back and forth - she's very nice, she's like my grandmother (in this life) Ella, taking care of me. Totally devoted to me, transfixed on my face. The other woman is like a cigar store Indian, making sure that everything is copacetic. It seems the woman rocking me is my grandmother.

Do you have any family?
I have a sister.

Let's go to a time when Alfred is older. Let's go to when Alfred is enjoying a meal.
Enjoying a meal, sitting in a pub, 24 now. Having a beer and some fish and chips. There are people in the pub, can't decipher what they're saying, they're wearing top hats. Like an Oxford club.

How are you feeling?
Concerned. Like there's a war that's going to start and I'm one of the guys who's going to have responsibility for some of the maneuvers.

Tell me about the people you work with.
It seems I've got on an army uniform, but with a beret; I'm older, in my 50's or 60's, very military like. It's the life of a loner, but I see it's been very hard for me to be in a relationship with people.

Let's go back to 24 years old... Back in the pub.
There's a war going on and I have to get the papers from England to France before the attack.

What's your last name?
H.. A..yden.. Alfred Hayden.

When you're 24 and there's a war brewing. What year is it?
1868.[58]

Let's go to when you're wearing your beret.
I'm outside, standing in front of an entire platoon of soldiers and I have a saber up against my chest, I have all these people in front of me and I'm about to address them. I'm in France.

As you address this platoon. What are you saying?
I'm trying to tell them we're going to be at war and we have to bond together and we're going to all have to put out the same energy and pay attention to what's going on and we'll win.

Ok, let's move forward to the last day of your life.
I've been shot in the chest. Two people behind me trying to revive me. Two women; one has me by the shoulders.

Are you inside?
No, I'm outside on the street, and I have a white shirt and blood is oozing out of my chest. I'm shot in the heart. I don't know who did it - they were looking for me.

What about the document?
I handed it over to the women, and said "Please hide this under your skirt." I'm lying down. I think this life had meaning and purpose; I was going to do something heroic.

NOTE: It's at the death scene that hypnotherapists can usually help the client see themselves in spirit form for the first time. It's usual that the first person they meet or experience in the life between lives is their spirit or soul guide, or guardian angel if you will.

---

[58] That would make his birth circa 1844. Alfred P. Hayden born in 1844 in MA from the 1880 census, Alfred G. Hayden born 1843 from Ohio, Alfred Hayden born 1845 in Essex, UK, Alfred Hayden born in 1843 in Wiltshire U.K.

A TRIP TO FIND HIS SOUL GUIDE

Let's float up and away from this life, looking down at your body… (etc).
I'm floating above. I'm in a chamber and there are three men, big powerful men with very big smiles on their faces, and there I am with some kind of document and they're going to stamp it and give me permission to be in the afterlife. As if to say "Oh here you are again, here's a pass. Have a good time." They're kind of laughing, "Why would you want to reincarnate again?" they say. "Aren't you having a good time up here with us? You can hang here with us; you can do whatever you want!" And they're happy to see me. And I feel happy to be with people who are happy to see me.

Is one of them sort of the main…?
One main one, kind of having this silent exchange with me.

How does he appear?
Big white robe, white beard. Jolly face. A fun red-faced, flushed. But he's big, must weigh five hundred pounds.

Tune into him. What's he saying to you?
"You're great, wonderful, look how talented you are, look what you did on Earth, you saved the entire French army, you've made people happy, you've sacrificed yourself. We're happy to have you up here, we hope you stay - we need somebody like you - selfless, we need you to help other people, bring them through and to guide them."

How's that feel?
I think it's my mission, here on Earth, to help people.

So he's happy with your performance in that life?
I'm a protector. I protect people; family, friends, animals, I'm concerned about you more than I am myself, I've always been that way, I'm a protector.

Would this gentleman answer some questions for us?
Yes, he's grabbed both my hands, I'm sitting on straw and he's sitting on a wooden bench. And we're going to have a dialog.

What's his name?
Let's call him Frenchie.

INTERVIEW WITH A SPIRIT GUIDE

I'd like to speak directly to Frenchie... Noel wants to ask you some questions... Number one is "why don't I feel like I fit in with most others?" Why does he feel that way?
Noel was beaten as a kid, had no self-esteem, and was told he was lousy, that nobody would ever marry him; that he was the cause of the divorce in his family. The reason he feels he doesn't fit in is because he's extra-sensory, he's more advanced on the enlightenment game than many people. He's very sensitive to feelings and takes them in as his own. He tries to give others love, light, to help their careers. He's a very funny person who wants to make everyone laugh and understand laughing and music are right next to godliness; you shouldn't be without them.

Is there some advice you can give him to transform the "no self-esteem" feelings?
He's doing what he can to transform himself.

Why did Noel choose this lifetime, when his birth father abandoned him?
To stand on his own two feet and not to rely on anyone. The other part was to protect his mother; once they're alone, he can shoulder the responsibility, protect her emotionally, physically, and financially.

What's the soul tie with Noel's mother? Why did he choose to become involved with her again?
To pay back a karma from some other time.

Show him in his mind, a picture of that scene or situation so he can understand.
We're in India. His mother is a dancer and what's coming out is that he killed her. And the payback is for her to kill him (emotionally) in this lifetime.

Why or how does he kill her? A lover? Friend? Stranger?
He killed her because she didn't love him. An Oedipal thing. She was a dancer and he thought she was cheap and she shouldn't be doing that because it was a religious family.

Are you in the same family?
I'm her father.

And she's dancing and you don't like that.
Because her sisters are doctors, her father's a judge, her mother's a nurse, what is she doing dancing? And she's dancing for a hound.

How does he kill her?
Stabs her with a knife.

Anything else he needs to know about his mother?
She's not done. She's coming back. She needs to have one good lifetime full of happiness. She had a very unhappy life. She'll have it (a happy one).

NOTE: Noel and his wife adopted a young girl from China. When the girl arrived, they both felt as if they'd known her for some time, as if she was meant to be in their lives. I encouraged Noel to bring some questions that he might want to have the hypnotherapist ask on his behalf, and one of them involved his adopted daughter Layla.

DID HE KNOW HIS ADOPTED DAUGHTER IN A PREVIOUS LIFE?

Is Layla, his daughter, known to him from another lifetime?
Layla is like his spirit guide, the most important person in his life. He's known her for many lifetimes. He's been dreaming about her for 50 years, "Where are you, when are you coming?"

She's like his spirit guide, what do you mean by that?
She is giving him the intuition to have a bigger and better life. Her presence is rejuvenating and exacting in terms of how he should be feeling. Part of it is that he's waited for her for so long. She's guided him to wait this long for her -- and now here she is.

In spirit, what is their relationship? Guide and student?
Soul mates. Layla has told him she's psychic.

Show him a lifetime on Earth together.
They were together on a Pacific island, they both have on loincloths and they're brother and sister, having a great time. They're having a picnic, there's a pool and a forest and it's beautiful there. Fruit for them to eat and they're just having a great time, being happy, being themselves. Living in paradise. Might have been Tahiti... Layla is Chinese, but in actuality she looks Polynesian as she did then.

What year was that?
1777.

Between then and now; any other lifetimes?
No. Just mental time.

Before Layla was born in this life did they have that mental connection?
Yes, there's a longing... when her face appeared in my mind's eye, I longed for her - "Come and be with me, show me your presence in my life," was the feeling.

What about Noel's issues with money?
I stole a bag of gold from the Emperor and got in his chariot. I was driving away, and he hit me in the side with a spear. I've been carrying around this pain for most of my life.

Let's talk to Frenchie about this.
Frenchie says "It's hard for him to accept the fact that he's done a beautiful job in this lifetime."

What does he need to know?
He has to be patient. There's no race against the clock to make money. Just hold on.

He wants to know "Can I conquer my fears, which are several..."
(Laughs.) He has so many fears; fear of dying, fear of flying, fear of being broke, fear of not being accepted, he has so many, he just has to forget about them. It's useless. Silly to put so much energy into it.

What's the best way to conquer the fears?
You just have to transmute the thought. The thought comes up and you can't fight the thoughts, but just let them pass, let them by. He's better at flying now.

Where did that fear originate?
He's not going to believe this... But it started in his mother's womb - something going on, having sex while she was pregnant, the bouncing, the turbulence shook him up.

What about the fear of dying?
It's less. With how I'm seeking and searching, I'm alleviating the fear.

What are you doing in the spiritual realm?
Learning. How to talk to people, the right dialogue, and the right way to interact with people. The right way to be aware of my surroundings.

How are you learning this?
Through my spiritual awareness.

You said that only 13% of your energy is here, and the other 87% is back in the life between lives... What is that energy doing back there? Any activities?
Only meditations and chartings.

What's your primary mission in this current life?
To make sure Layla has enough for herself when I'm gone and part of my mission is to make people happy, enjoy life, make them see and feel a rush of spirituality. How that would make them feel.

How about in terms of his own development?
For him to feel self-love. If he had self-love, none of the other things would really matter.

Anything else he needs to know?
Slow and steady, don't rush it.

NOTE: Noel's ensuing trip to his soul group seems to include his Council of Elders. According to Newton's research, soul groups are usually between 3 and 25 souls that we reincarnate with for millennia – sometimes they drop out and move upwards or laterally into other groups, and sometimes we find new ones in our group, depending on their level of progression. In the case of the Council, clients normally report a group of 6-12 non reincarnating individuals who appear for their benefit – not to judge them – but to help them understand the lessons from the previous life just lived.

THE SOUL GROUP

Frenchie, somewhere else you'd like to show your friend? Soul groups? Soul mates, library...
He's taken me into this vestibule that has rows of men and women sitting there and they have on white, looks like robes. And he's leading me, where I'm going to meet, I guess, someone.

Describe the scene for me...
Can you think of the plaza in front of the Vatican at Christmas? Lit, bright, like an atomic blast, bright in the room - everyone sitting very straight, magnificent, their expressions are very all-knowing and powerful and Frenchie has me by the left hand and is looking at them and looking at me as if to say "Look, look at all these people you have around you who are going to maybe give you some tender love and care."

How do you feel going in there?
I'm always suspicious about love... And authority - but I feel pretty good. This is awe inspiring.

About how many beings are there?
Thirty-six. Three rows of twelve. Male and female. Oh, there's a friend of mine, Lorenzo. He was a client of mine who shot himself two weeks ago, because he had money problems and couldn't face them; he was depressed. He's come forward and he's looking at me and is mentally passing these thoughts to me; "Don't do what I did. Doesn't make sense. Don't be depressed." and then "You don't have to compare yourself to me or anybody in this room."

"That's been your problem," Frenchie says. "Comparing yourself to everyone in this room. You know you shouldn't." That's what Lorenzo is telling me as well; "don't compare."

Is Lorenzo okay?
He's happy; he's in the middle of the 36 people. He was a really dear friend. He's okay.

Can you maintain a connection with him?
I always will. His artwork is all over my house. He's an artist.

Does he feel like he made a mistake?
In truth he feels he did the right thing, because in his death his art is going to be much more valuable for his family. It's an awful tragedy. I wish he hadn't. I had no idea he was so depressed.

Describe this place for me.
Pristine, white, immaculate.

Let's talk about the life you left as Alfred for a moment.
I was a hero. I was like The Scarlet Pimpernel; major espionage guy. I was highly thought of, had an enormous home in London with butlers, maids; but I led a double life, which was the life of a spy. Which is really interesting because in Noel's real life he represents some people in the espionage world and police world - and he wonders "why do they come to him?" It's not like he has a few, he has many. So that life is playing out in this life somehow.

NOTE: In Noel's life as a successful media executive, he's frequently in contact with authors and others who bring him literary works – during his lifetime he's worked with a number of famous authors who had lives in the CIA and espionage world.

THE COUNCIL OF ELDERS

Let's talk to the council about your current state. How's he doing?
In unison they're saying he's doing just great, we don't know many people who can do the kind of work he's doing and have the spiritual path he's on. He needs a pat on the back, and he's been told he's got a life in spirit. Teaching spiritualism is something he's good at and he should do it - he's giving yoga classes at his house and he's into many Eastern spiritual teachers.

Why did he choose his rough childhood?
What's coming up is that he's going to achieve the life he wants because he needed to struggle. He had success in past lives, but in this one, he needed to become aware. He will be more fulfilled; he's at the precipice of awareness. We've just got to tell him to keep doing what he's doing. He's doing okay.

Can I ask the council about Layla?
They're no two people more bonded in the universe than Noel and his daughter. She's the light of his life, every day she teaches him something and he's ready to learn. He wasn't before, but he is now.

Any other members of the council that want to give you a message?
There was a woman in my life who said I got her pregnant and I denied it and a few weeks later she killed herself. I've always felt responsible and she's on my council and has come forward to tell me to stop feeling guilty. I didn't kill her, she killed herself. I'm to stop feeling guilty about it.

I'd like to ask a question to the council. Why has he been brought to this session today?
He needs to imprint the phenomenon that there are past lives and he does have guides, and he does have protection for himself and has council members that will talk to him.

To sum up, what's the purpose of this session today?
To experience, to figure if he wants to go further in this field and to also bring as much light and intelligence and love back to his daughter and back to his wife.

Anyone else on the council?
Yes, I see my grandmother. (A pause, while he speaks to her) Okay.

Etch this in your mind, the bright light, and the loving people. Is there somewhere else Frenchie would like to guide you to?
NOTE: In Noel's council, or soul group, he was able to see a number of close friends and relatives. He saw a friend who had recently committed suicide, and after the session told the man's widow about seeing him. He also saw his grandmother there, someone who'd always given him unconditional love. However, it's the next episode that is unique to Noel in my research – from all the good works that he's done in his lifetimes, cathedrals have been built in his honor. According to Frenchie, both have been constructed out of the good deeds that he's done in his lifetime; one secular, and one religious. Noel grew up Jewish, I found it interesting for him to describe a soaring Cathedral as one of his "intention created" palaces.

TWO CATHEDRALS BUILT FROM INTENTIONS

Frenchie wants to bring me to a gigantic church with 100 foot ceilings, gold statues, pews made of gold, tremendous choir singing, just the two of us, sitting and listening - the whole thing is for us...

What is this place?
He says "This is your church, this is your synagogue and this is your temple, I just want to show you that all the spiritual things you're doing right... It's your holy

place. Your church, temple, synagogue, ashram. We've built it for you."

You've helped build it with your devotions?
Right. Frenchie's leading me to a different place that looks like the Taj Mahal and he says "Come in, this is yours too. (Gestures with his hands) That's yours and this is yours, you deserve it and you've earned it, it comes with servants and elephants and monkeys and food and wine and fruit and you can have six wives or seven mistresses, or none, and there's children and food and people are happy in this Taj Mahal; it's yours." It's huge.

So you have this as well.
He's got his spirit and his secular; it's been built with your spirit and they're both enormous benefits to you - walk into the church to feel the energy or bring people into the Taj Mahal, give them gold, whatever you want in an endless supply. And Frenchie says, "You can come back here anytime you want, they're never going to go away, they're yours forever."

Awesome. Maybe it's time to rest... Let's have Frenchie take you somewhere to do that.
We're in Tahiti in a grass hut and I'm on this table and I'm being massaged and oiled and my shoulders are being rubbed and it's just a beautiful Tahitian breeze and it's wonderful and so relaxing and then as soon as they're done I'm going into a deep sleep and relaxing; they've given me something to drink; some kind of relaxing tea.

Let's ask Frenchie about the kidney problem you mentioned...
I asked (my doctors) for an operation to fix it, they wouldn't do it. They said "Let's live with it."

Let's ask Frenchie. Is there a deeper meaning?
The one that keeps coming up is the spear in the side - I was running away and they got me.

So what's the message you're supposed to get?
That you can't run away from yourself. That truth is your identity and if you live the truth then anything aberrant or off to the side is going to dissipate. That's the best you can do.

So once again...
"Don't run away from the truth. Because if you run away, we're going to throw another spear at you." It's like saying "Take what belongs to you and don't run away from it." You didn't need to steal the gold, it was yours, you were the son of the King, and it was your gold. Why were you stealing it?"

The spear in the back, you understand it now?
It feels better already.

Okay, keep your church and the Taj Mahal close to your heart... (Etc as Scott talks Noel back to consciousness)."
Afterwards, Noel told me about his lifelong problem with his kidney, that he could never sit for more than a few minutes without being in pain. Doctors had diagnosed a faulty flap on his kidney, but after the session he claimed that the pain was gone. When I asked him the following week about it, he said, "It feels like an echo of a pain that used to be there. I'd say it's 95% gone now." I spoke to his Doctor recently, and he said when Noel came to see him, according to his blood tests, he was close to renal failure. His lifelong issue with pain from his kidney was causing his kidneys to fail. After his past life regression and dealing with the issues underlying the pain, (and combined with care that his Doctor was giving him) Noel had this amazing revelation. His recent blood tests show his kidneys are back to normal. A 100% complete, verifiable recovery. His Doctor told me "I've never seen this quick a recovery of any patient that had the kind of kidney problems Noel had. He went from blood tests that showed clearly he was on the brink of renal failure, to being *100% normal.*" His Doctor credited his Past Life regression as the catalyst for the dramatic recovery.

Recently Noel attended a yoga class with a well-known psychic who began a reading by asking "The name Alfred is coming to me that has something to do with the military. Is there anyone here with a connection to the military named Alfred?" Noel was surprised to hear the name and occupation of his past life persona; he'd only learned it the previous night.

In terms of his adoption of his daughter; Noel said he had dreams of a Polynesian woman's face for most of his life. It wasn't until the adoption of Layla that he recognized her as the person he'd been dreaming about. And even though Layla was adopted from an orphanage in China, as she's grown older, her looks have become decidedly Polynesian.

As I said to Noel, who would have known that we'd become friends 30 years ago so I could introduce him to the Doctor and Hypnotherapist who would cure his kidney ailment that I had no idea about. Is it possible that moves on the chess board of our lives are planned years, decades in advance? What this research shows is that not only are our choices of lives pre-planned on some level, but our parent's journey as well. And by logical extension, our parents' parents' journey. If that's the case, then how far back does the thread run?

"The only real voyage of discovery consists not in seeking new landscapes but in having new eyes."

- Marcel Proust

Chapter 13
DAD'S ON THE PHONE

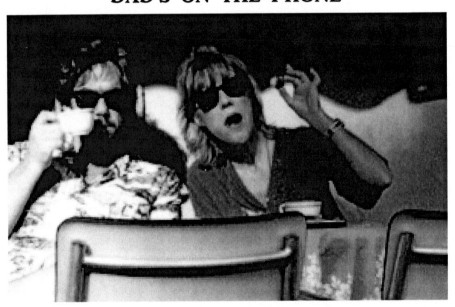

"The extent to which scientists are uninformed about the real work of nonscientists seems to me to reach some ultimate point when scientists consider meditative states, alterations in consciousness, and the disputed psychic phenomena. If you have never experienced these things firsthand, you will naturally find the descriptions of them to be outlandish."

- Michael Crichton[59]

---

[59] "Travels" Michael Crichton's autobiography of 1988.

"Monique" is a model and a successful actress in New York, has appeared on a number of Soap Operas, and has a number of internet sites dedicated to her. She had no experience with talking to people in the afterlife, but her father committed suicide when she was a young girl, and it was something she rarely mentioned to anyone. Recently married, the 20 something actress received an odd phone call from John Edward, the psychic.

He wanted to know if she could come into his office in Long Island and speak to him about something important. John claimed that during a session with another client, her father had suddenly come through, and had convinced him to track her down through the Screen Actors Guild. Wary at first, she brought her then fiancée with her to visit Edward's office on Long Island. She'd never seen his show, nor knew anyone who'd met him. Once inside his office, he apologized for the odd form of introduction, and quickly went about his work of bringing her father into the room.

Monique didn't know what to think, her father's death wasn't something she spoke of, and didn't believe it to be public knowledge. John said her father was asking if she'd make a phone call to her mother, who lived in Michigan. Monique picked up the phone and called her mother, saying "Mom, you'll never guess where I am." The mother was familiar with Edward's show, and was surprised to be getting a call from the afterlife from her deceased husband.

Through Edward, the father asked Monique's mom to "go downstairs, there's something he wants you to find." The mother went downstairs with her cordless portable phone. "Okay, I'm downstairs," she said. John said her father wanted her to search for a red folder - a book filled with family photographs, that she would find on a shelf in the back bedroom downstairs. According to Monique, she listened as John directed the mother past other rooms, specifically telling her which direction to turn.

The mother followed his instructions and found the folder. She pulled it from its perch on a dusty shelf and opened it up to find family pictures - pictures taken when the father was healthy, not depressed - a time when he was happiest. John said that the father "Wants you to look at those photographs and remember him as he once was - because as he was then in those pictures, happy and carefree, he is now. He's no longer filled with sadness or depression, and wants you to know how much he loves you."

The mother and Monique were both in tears. John added that the father was saying that Monique was pregnant, or about to be so, which came as a surprise to her and her fiancée. That particular detail turned out to be true as well, and she's now the proud mom of a baby boy, and happy to have made a connection with her father so long after his passing. She told me she'd never sought out a psychic to reach out to her father. The only rational explanation for John Edward to call her, reach out to her mother, direct her to find the family photo album, was if the father was actually speaking from beyond the grave.

According to James Van Praagh in "Talking to Heaven," the photographs of loved ones are frequent places that resonate energy. He recounts a number of sessions where the deceased says their loved one was "standing in front of my photograph" when they remember some moment in their lives. There's a section where Van Praagh claims that if a subject meditates on a photograph of a loved one, or the object once held or owned or worn by a loved one, with a specific question for that loved one, the loved one will find a way to reply. It might be through a phone call from a friend, or some other incident that on the face of it seems coincidental.

My first experience with a psychic was after Luana passed away, I was working with our mutual friend, the actor, comedian, political wit and social activist Charles Grodin. I was occasionally appearing on his show as a correspondent out in Los Angeles when I saw the psychic James Van Praagh on Larry King, and discussed with Charles bringing him on his show. Charles is skeptical about hearing from people in the Great Beyond, but eventually asked him to appear on the show. He then arranged for me to be a caller - no one on the staff knew I was going to call in, James Van Praagh didn't know me, or that I'd be calling in. It was Charles' own way of performing a test for his guest without his knowledge.

I said Luana's name, and Van Praagh began describing her death in accurate detail, my sitting at her bedside and holding her hand - her sudden departure from breast cancer. He said that he could hear that she had a terrific laugh, and said "She's laughing about a cocktail glass collection that you have in your kitchen." I have a collection of Martini glasses people have given me because of my last name. He then said "She says there's a photograph on your refrigerator that's the essence of your relationship." I thought that was pretty uncanny. I can only remember once in my life speaking out loud to a photograph, and it was when I put the photo of me and Luana on my refrigerator. We're sitting in Rome together, at a cafe. I had set the self-timer on the camera and returned to our table and lifted up my cappuccino. Luana was snacking on a croissant and laughing, holding her fingers up as if to say "How tasty!" As I tacked it onto my fridge, I said aloud "Well, there's the essence of our relationship; laughter and cappuccino." So when Van Praagh said those words, a shiver went up my spine. A few minutes later, I said "Thank you," and he said "And remember, when you feel that shiver go up your spine, she's telling you you're on the right track."

My father was diagnosed with Alzheimer's when he was in his early 80's. It was a slow and difficult process, and I tried to visit him and my mom in our Chicago suburban home every couple of months or so. I would go home and shave him, or tell him stories, always trying to make sure I included him in conversations - even though his outward appearance didn't seem to show that he was paying attention, I always remember what someone told me about the process; "He may not remember who you are, but you remember who he is."

I was in Los Angeles the day he passed away. I knew he'd been confined to his bed a couple of days, and in my prayers for him the night before, I prayed for him to "let go." When the phone rang in the morning, I knew what the news would be and booked myself the earliest flight home. By nightfall I was back at the house he designed and built for his family. I consoled my mom, and like the Irish/Italian family we are, spent time reminiscing with my three brothers over glasses of wine.

As I lay in bed that night, I awoke to feel a hand on my shoulder. I knew it was his hand before I even woke up. I said in my head "Dad, how are you?" And he responded, in my ear, "I'm experiencing indescribable joy." It's not the kind of thing I'd ever heard him say before, and was startled to hear his voice so clear, as he hadn't been able to speak clearly the past few years. The next morning I asked my mother about it - "Do you remember dad ever saying something was indescribably beautiful?" She said yes, rarely, and usually when he couldn't find the words to describe the beauty he was seeing.

Then that following night, he woke me again. This time, I could hear him walking down our hallway - the floor creaked, he had a particular walk - I knew it was him, and could feel his presence in my bedroom. After a pause I heard him say clearly in my ear; "I need you to write something down."

Of course, part of me was saying "Is that really him talking, or am I imagining this?" So I paused a second and said to myself "Just tell me what it is, I'll remember it in the morning." Another pause. "I need you to write something down." I was awake now, and what the hell was I doing arguing with my dad's spirit anyways? I put on the light, took a piece of paper and pencil, then turned off the light, with the moon out the window giving me enough light to see, I raised my pencil.

He said "Tell your mother I love her very much. Tell her that I'm here with Ma and Pa (his parents) Velia and Rig (his brother and sister) and Harry." He named other people, I wrote their names down, but I had no idea who they were. He said "It's beautiful here. I love you." Then he said "I need you to write a note for each of your brothers." I picked up a piece of paper and he dictated three different notes - each one specifically tailored to each brother. I finally asked in my mind's eye; "So why are you telling me this stuff?" He answered "Because you can hear me."

Sometime later, after my daughter was two, and her brother was born, my wife and I were sitting in the living room watching television. Olivia came in from the kitchen with her eyes wide. "Grandpa's in the kitchen." I didn't move, but looked at my wife. "Why do you think he's here?" Olivia looked over at her baby brother in her mother's arms. "To see the baby!" I chuckled, and then asked if there was anything Grandpa wanted to say to us. "He says I love you," she said, in her little two year old voice. Then she looked around the living room of our apartment - a room filled with toys for the two kids. "He says you guys need a bigger home." My wife and I laughed. That would definitely be something my father the architect would say.

One other story about my father and the energy of his work; on two separate occasions I was in the room where I felt his presence - before he'd passed away. Once was when I was at La Fonda Hotel in Santa Fe, New Mexico. I was standing in the lobby, and had an overwhelming sense of him in the room. I walked over to the pay phone and called him. I asked "Dad, why am I sensing you here at La Fonda Hotel in Santa Fe?" He said "Maybe because I designed the interior when I worked for Holabird and Root in Chicago." That was the prestigious architectural firm he began his career with in my home town.

The other time was when I was in Luana's home in Mar Vista, California. It was a small Craftsman with one bedroom, and she'd had another bedroom built which had lots of light. I was sitting on the bed in the new extension when I suddenly said "Oh my god. This is my father's room." She said, "I told you I asked your dad to do some drawings for me." In my blockheadedness, I hadn't realized that drawings meant designs - it was his design, and I could literally sense his presence in the room from the way the light came through the windows, or the lines of the room. All I can say is that when I am in a room that my father designed, I can feel it. Could a person's *intent* stay with their creative work of art?

Michael Crichton trained as a Harvard doctor, and then began writing novels and screenplays; "The Andromeda Strain" and "Jurassic Park" are among his most famous. He also created the show "ER." His journey through life included exploration of psychic phenomena, and although never fully convinced of its veracity, he pursued it throughout his adult life through therapy and hypnotherapy. Despite being trained in traditional medicine, he was surprisingly open to different modalities. I found the following passage in his book, and am reproducing it here, because despite been written about 8 years before Michael Newton published his first book, you'll see the similarities with the other past life regressions. The past life regression is reprinted from Michael Crichton's book "Travels." It was not offered in the book as an accurate past life regression, nor was it given any spiritual weight other than "This odd psychic event happened to me." It bears repeating because in light of this research, he had the same kind of regression that many people do, and wasn't able to see the connection between his past life as a Gladiator, and his present one as an Author.

Past life regression with friend and hypnotist *Gary* and Michael Crichton[60]

Gary: What's going on?
Michael: I'm in Rome. I smell the odors of the arena, blood and sand and animal excrement. Above me I hear the roar of the crowd, the stomping feet. I feel the heat of the day in my tiny, oppressive cell as I wait.

Where in Rome?
The Coliseum.

[60] "Travels" by Michael Crichton. Published by Alfred A. Knopf 1988. Pgs 305-308. I've taken the liberty of putting his words into present tense to maintain the transcription style of this book.

How does it feel?
I'm very strong. I'm aware of my enormous body, my great physical strength. I am startled to feel genuine pleasure at having a large body, to feel proud of it and not to be embarrassed by it, as I am in real life. Here in the Coliseum, I need this body; I need to rely on it. But this is also a different body, hard, heavily muscled, and dark-skinned. And I feel something else - a sick, tense feeling, anxiety. Adrenaline. I have to kill people; kill them before they kill me.

How does that feel?
It doesn't matter, I have to do it or I will be killed. I have to kill them first. It is my job.

Do you know the people you are fighting?
I don't want to know them. I may have to kill them. I'm not afraid to die.

How many people have you killed?
It... doesn't matter.

It doesn't sound like a very nice life. Do you have women?
Sometimes. They supply women to the fighters. Prostitutes. Hard women. Sometimes rich women come to amuse themselves.

How do you feel about the women?
I have no feeling. Here in Rome I feel nothing except my size and my strength and my certainty that I will win. There's nothing else to feel; there's no room for anything else.

That must not be pleasant, to have no feelings.
There's nothing wrong with me. I've been a gladiator all my life. I was a slave in Tunisia, I was sent to Rome and I grew so large I was sold as a gladiator. I have won many fights. I am nineteen; I have lived that long.

What will happen to you?
I will die. By lion.

How do you feel about that death?
I have no feeling. It's an encounter, fatigue, a mistake, nothing more. There is nothing to have feeling about. It is just animal interaction; two animals together.

What do you think of your life as a gladiator?
I'm not going to talk to you anymore.

That ended Michael's past life regression. He told his friend and hypnotist Gary that he believed because he's a writer he'd made the entire episode up. This is the common feeling people have when they reconnect with their conscious mind after a session; "I must have made the whole thing up." Crichton says he was

143

comfortable with his height and weight as a Gladiator, as opposed to how tall he was in this life – but wasn't able to see how the energy that he brought into film and television world required a Gladiator mentality; there's a connection between the two. Generally when people have a past life memory, it's a life that has some connection with their current one.

I arranged for a prolific reality television Producer to have a past life regression in New York City with Paul Aurand. During the session, he clearly remembered a life in Wales where he was the daughter of a King, or Chieftain who was disappointed in having a daughter. He said after the father's death, he saw himself gathering the troops and leading them into battle, where she saw herself riding through the fog into soldiers, and being impaled through her armor onto one of their spears.

What the reality TV producer hadn't considered until I asked him; how does that relate to this life? Do you have any issues with your father about why you chose your profession? Is there a sense of disappointment you're trying to overcome? It then became clear to him why he'd had the past life memory of the King's daughter. True or not, the remembering of it helps us in this lifetime.

There's a later episode in "Travels" that appears to represent a "life between life" moment with Crichton's father with whom he reported having a difficult relationship. Here's his description of his out-of-body experience meeting his father "on an astral plane" during a guided meditation, again with his close friend and hypnotist *Gary*.

Gary: How do you feel?
Michael: I appear to be in a misty yellow place. I begin to see why people imagine heaven as misty or cloudy. It's peaceful to be standing in this yellow mist. I feel fine.

Do you see anybody here?
No.

Stay there a minute and let's see if anybody comes.

I see my grandmother who died while I was in medical school. She waves to me and I wave back. I'm not surprised to see her here. I don't feel any particular need to talk to her.

Do you see anybody else?
Yes. My father. He approaches me; he looks the same, only translucent and misty. I'm nervous. He's embracing me. In that instant, I see and feel everything in my relationship with my father, all the feelings he has and why he found me difficult, all the feelings I have and why I misunderstood him, all the love that is between us, and all the confusion and misunderstanding that overpowered it. I see all the things he has done for me and all the ways he's helped me. I see every aspect of our relationship at once. It was an instant of compassionate acceptance and love. He's hugging me.

What are you feeling?
The incredibly powerful experience was complete and total in a fraction of a second. My relationship with my father has been resolved in a flash."

This is a common experience in a session through an embrace; two souls experience all the feelings and emotions the other person had during their lifetime. They experience everything you experienced in your lifetime, and you experience theirs. The feeling is reportedly to be pure bliss to be able to understand another person so deeply, as well as healing for all wounds; one has the opportunity to see and feel the negative thoughts they had about a person, and with the embrace, wash them all away.

Michael Crichton passed away in 2008. The energy he put into his books, his screenplays, his directing – all of that still exists, accessible not only in celluloid, but lives on in all of us who have experienced his writing, his vision, his mind.

We've all heard about famous last words, the last utterances of famous and the infamous. Is it possible that last words are actually the first words being said in the next life?

"It's so silly. All you do is get the heck out of your body when you die. My gosh, everybody's done it thousands of times. Just because they don't remember, it doesn't mean they haven't done it."

- J D Salinger

CHAPTER 14
FAMOUS LAST WORDS

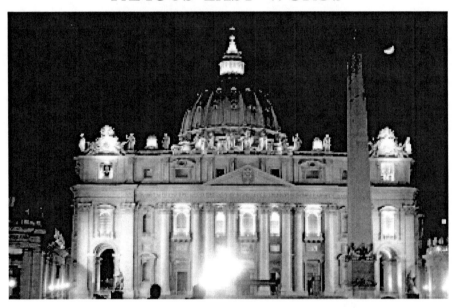

"It's very beautiful over there." - Thomas Edison
"I should never have switched from Scotch to Martinis." - Humphrey Bogart
"Why not? Why not? Why not? Beautiful." - Timothy Leary
"I'm tired of fighting. I guess this thing is going to get me." - Harry Houdini
"Everything is an illusion." - Mata Hari
"Dying is easy, comedy is hard." - George Bernard Shaw
"Curtain! Fast music! Light! Great! The show looks good!" - Florenz Ziegfeld
"France. The Army. Head of the Army. Josephine!" - Napoleon
"Ha. Ha. Ha." - Luana Anders

Napoleon's last words sound as if he was reporting for duty, then saw his long lost love: "France. The Army. Head of the Army… Josephine!" Napoleon was fond of telling his generals he believed in reincarnation and who he was in a past life. So perhaps he's merely reporting for duty in the life between lives.

Magician Harry Houdini had an experience doing a stunt that famously changed his life. While performing an escape from a frozen river, he became trapped under the ice. He heard his dead mother's voice telling him where the escape route was, and through her guidance found the way out. Afterwards, he went to many well-known psychics to see if he could contact his mother again. He spent the rest of his days debunking these charlatans, proving they were manufacturing results and playing with people's fantasies in order to gain fortune and notoriety. He was unable to reach his mother again.

In Dr. Jeffrey Long's study of Near Death Experiences (NDE's), "Evidence of the Afterlife," he recounts a patient Ramona whose brother-in-law Bob died in 2000. Bob had been watching the film "Houdini" with his wife Marsha which covered the part of the famous magician's search to find his mother. Bob didn't believe in the afterlife, so he and his wife came up with an obscure phrase that one would pass along to the other if there was life after death. Sometime after he died, Ramona had the uncontrollable urge to call Marsha and say "Yellow bubbles," – indeed, it was the secret phrase Marsha and Bob had created - something so obscure they knew no one would ever randomly say it.[61]

Alaska Flight 261 crashed off the California coast in 2000 and as they were bringing up effects from the ocean floor using a steel cage, a worker noticed a ring on the deck of the ship. It belonged to Bob Williams, 65, who died with his wife Patty, 63 in the crash. However, his daughter Tracy Knizek believed the ring was a sign from her father.[62] "Ever since I was a little girl, my dad and I had a deal," she said. "Whoever died first, the other one would come back and tell them what it's like. It was just to let the other person know if it's OK, like we think it's going to be. I knew me and my brothers were going to be OK."[63]

What's going on here? Wish fulfillment? Or something deeper? Many stories of the spirit world can be summed up with "It may have happened to one person, but can't be replicated." Personal tales of near death experiences, NDE's, messages from the departed, or even channeling fall into this "first person account" category. Scientists have shown a particular part of the brain is activated during a near death experience, or an out of body experience, and use that to explain why a person might imagine they're experiencing things outside of themselves when their brain scan shows they really aren't.

There've been studies done of out of body experiences during operations, where doctors have placed written words on top of lamps, so if a patient has an

[61] Pg 191 "Evidence of the Afterlife" by Jeffrey Long, MD with Paul Perry. Harper One 2010
[62] "The Crash of Flight 261" LA Times, Feb 6, 2000
[63] Newsday, Feb 4th, 2000. "Crash Victim's Ring Spurs Conflict."

OBE, they can report what they saw during the operation.[64] There are many who claim to be standing next to their body during surgery, observing what the doctors are doing, or in some cases, not doing, and report those observations. In Deepak Chopra's "Life After Death," he says he knew a doctor who walked into a room as a patient was dying and saw a ghostly like energy rise up out of the dead man.[65] There are cases where people feel like they're dead and somewhere during their journey, return because "I wasn't ready to go," or "They pulled me back here."[66]

Dr. Kenneth Ring, a psychologist and professor Emeritus at the University of Connecticut is one of the foremost researchers on Near Death Experiences and has catalogued hundreds. In a discussion with parapsychologist Jeffrey Mishlove, Dr. Ring talked about people who experience a full life review while having an NDE, when they see their "life flash before my eyes." In his book "Lessons from the Light," he reports about blind people who see and identify objects during a NDE that are confirmed independently.[67] He claims people become "Less materialistic, more spiritually orientated, and discover psychic gifts that weren't present before, but develop as a result," after a near-death experience.

"It isn't just a life review," he says, "it's a re-living of your life, when people are able to describe every single act that you have ever done, every single thought, every single word that you have spoken, suddenly, all of this is back with you. You run through it again, you see and experience the effects of these thoughts, acts and words with other people." One example he gives:

"I have a friend who had a hot temper, and one day he was driving in his hometown, and almost ran someone over. Angry at the pedestrian, he punched him out, got back into his truck and roared off. Fifteen years later, he had an NDE, had a 'life review' and this scene came up - he said he re-experienced the event as if viewing events from above, but also in the role of the pedestrian; he felt all 32 blows inflicted on himself, his teeth cracking, tasting the blood in the mouth, a complete role reversal. This is the sort of thing people report; in our life review we become the people we hurt and also those we helped feel good. When people talk about "The Golden Rule" in the context of the NDE, it's the way of the Universe and you experience this during the life review. That's why people change as much as they do after having one. To see everything you've ever done is a heavy lesson that stays with you."[68]

---

[64] "Mortal Minds: Biology of Near Death" by G. M. Woerlee

[65] "Life After Death" by Deepak Chopra. The book claims the soul's trajectory "is always upwards" which follows the Hindu concept of Karma and how lives are chosen for us because of it. However, this research shows people volunteer for "lesser" or more difficult lives in order to progress more fully in the spirit realm; there is no trajectory for souls, only compassionate choices.

[66] "Evidence of the Afterlife." Ibid.

[67] http://video.google.com/videoplay?docid=-1926194465658058884#

[68] Ibid.

During the Iraq war, the L.A. Times did a feature article about a soldier who appeared in a photo smoking a cigarette, strikingly handsome, a dirty face, he was dubbed "The Marlboro Man" by the media. Some years later, the photographer found this Marine suffering from post-traumatic stress, living in a trailer, having lost his wife due to his violent flashbacks from when he was a sniper in Iraq.

The Marine talked about his job; "To try to live with that... how do you justify it, regardless of what your causes are or what their causes are?" he said. "To see somebody in your sights and to pull that trigger... (to) see their life flash before (your) eyes as well as taking it. It's an insane connection you make with that person at that point."[69]

Under hypnosis, people often claim their death in a previous lifetime was part of a contract or an agreement to go through a particular experience. The victims may have already known the person who was going to take their lives, and in some cases, not only knew it, but asked the other person to perform this task so that they could learn a spiritual lesson from it.

Former Time/Warner President Gerald Levin's son was murdered in a senseless crime while teaching underprivileged children in the Bronx. Later, Gerald's soon to be new wife, Laurie, who is psychic, told Gerald his son had spoken to her and said he'd agreed to be murdered in such a dramatic way so his father could help other people by setting up clinics for children in underprivileged high schools.[70]

A senseless death in this life may make sense in the life between lives.

Sam Kinison was a gregarious comic in the 1980's when he had a tragic car accident on his way to a gig in Vegas. It's been widely reported when he got out of the car, laid down on the ground, he looked up as if speaking to someone. According to eyewitness Carl LaBove, Sam said "No, no, I don't want to die." Sam paused, as if listening to a voice. "But why?" he asked. LaBove said it sounded as if he was having a conversation. "Then I heard him go, "Ok, ok, ok." The last "Ok' was so soft and at peace, like he was talking to someone he loved."[71]

There are many familial stories of people on their death bed seeing other people in their room, departed loved ones, or strangers. Sometimes the departing ones return for a few moments of lucidity to say something profound to their loved ones about what's on the other side; its beauty, or what awaits them.

A close friend of Luana was battling cancer recently and spent six months in the hospital. She was medicated much of the time, but told me that a young handsome man would come in every day and tell her stories and make her laugh. She called him the "Jazz Man" because they talked about jazz and other things. He was light and funny, and she looked forward to his visits. And then one day some of her friends came and sat with her, and she was eager to introduce her new friend to

[69] LA Times. "The Marlboro Marine." By Luis Sinco. Nov. 12, 2007
[70] "God, the Universe, and Where I Fit In: A Psychic's Reflections on Figuring Out the Rest of Your Life" by Laurie Ann Levin
[71] LA Times, "Friends Shocked by Violent Death of Mellower Kinison" by Amy Wallace. April 12, 1992.

them... And at some point during the introduction, noting their reaction, she said "You can't see him, can you?" The young man smiled at her and eventually melted away. Instrumental in bringing her back to health, she has no idea who he was.

There's a great story about how "It's a Wonderful Life" was conceived by Frank Capra. In his book "Name Above The Title[72]" Capra recounts how after he won the Oscar for "It Happened One Night," he went into a depression, fearing he wouldn't be able to recreate his success. He began telling people he didn't want to see them because he "wasn't feeling well," and after making up the excuse so many times, he actually didn't feel well. He was confined to a bed, and every doctor that came to see him couldn't figure out what his malady was, but were convinced, perhaps by Mr. Capra, that he really was dying.

And then one day, a short bald man came into his room and berated the famous film director for pretending to be sick. He told him he was acting like a child, that he owed it to his audience to get out of bed and make films; he could help people with his talent, and he was wasting it by hiding in bed. The iconic director said that after the man left, everyone said they didn't see the stranger, and no one could tell him who he was. He called up his writing partner, Albert Hackett, forced himself into a car, and they drove to a desert resort where they wrote "It's A Wonderful Life" together.[73] Whoever sent the stranger; thank you.

And seeing ghosts aren't limited to single cases. Arthur C. Clarke, author of "2001 – a Space Odyssey," hosted a television show called "Mysterious Universe," where he would debunk paranormal tales. In one incident, a couple went to Versailles and when they crossed a bridge saw a crowd of people wearing wigs, looking every bit as if from the past. When they asked about the "re-enactment" they were told there wasn't any; the couple accurately described Versailles as it had been before a renovation. In another case, two English tourists got lost while traveling during a storm, and checked into a small hotel for the night. The next day, they went to retrieve a suitcase left behind and were told their hotel had burned down during World War II. Clarke said he couldn't dismiss their claims, and could only chalk them up to some kind of "group hypnosis." This same phenomenon has been reported near Gettysburg, where tourists occasionally claim to witness soldiers marching in formation, and then disappear into a mist.

A psychologist told me a story of how her friend's disabled daughter had wandered off one stormy night into a forest near their vacation cabin. The frantic family got a call from a waitress at a restaurant; the daughter was safe and was ready to be picked up. The mother drove into the rainstorm and picked up her daughter – but when she returned a few days later to thank the staff, she learned the restaurant had burned down some years before.

Even in my family, my mother talks about the day she lost my older brother. Jeff

---

[72] Capra, Frank. *Frank Capra, The Name Above the Title: An Autobiography.* Macmillan, 1971.

[73] Francis Frances Goodrich, Albert Hackett and Frank Capra are the official writers on the film, however Jo Swerling, Philip Van Doren Stern wrote the story.

had wandered off, and she was trying to find him when an elderly Priest with white hair dropped him at home. The Priest told her the parish he was with and how he'd found my brother in the pews. The next day she called the Church to thank him; the Parish claimed no such Priest was serving there.

Then there are people who predict their own deaths, or predict other calamities about to befall them. After the 1984 Olympics, John Dupont, heir to the family fortune, hired Olympic Gold Medalist Dave Schultz to teach him to wrestle. Dupont was unbalanced however, and at some point killed the young Olympian. At his son's funeral, Dave's father revealed something his son had told him that predicted his death. He said while they were walking in the woods behind their home, his five year old son had asked him if he could keep a secret. The father said "Ok." His son said "Before I came here I went to the council and they agreed I could come here to teach a lesson in love. But I won't be here very long." [74]

It was that statement that came back to haunt the father after his son's death, but also comforted him in an odd way - his son knew he wouldn't be here for "very long." According to this research, we make two trips to this august council; once when we return, to help us examine the life just lived, and again before departure to this realm, where we reconfirm why we're making this choice of a lifetime. But it wasn't until a close friend lost his daughter that I realized this form of therapy could actually help in the healing process from a terrible loss.

Death ends a life, not a relationship.

- Jack Lemmon

---

[74] Carol Bowman "Children's Past Lives." and Unsolved Mysteries, Gettysburg Ghosts, Season 1, Episode 4.

CHAPTER 15
OUT OF THE BLUE

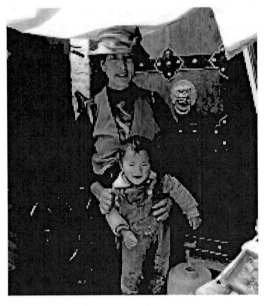

"Would you know my name, if I saw you in heaven? Will it be the same, if I saw you in heaven?"

-Eric Clapton[75]

---

[75] "Tears In Heaven" words and music by Eric Clapton and Will Jennings

A phone call came for me out of the blue. I was on a film set in Venice, California, filming bookends for a Bollywood film called "My Faraway Bride," when I got a call from an old friend from Chicago. I hadn't spoken to Chuck Tebbets since our last day in high school in Northbrook, Illinois, bucolic home to Olympic skater Ann Henning and prolific filmmaker John Hughes.

Chuck designed a website for the Tibetan government in exile, and discovered I had a connection to the Tibetan people through my documentary work.[76] He called because he wanted me to come to London and help him create a web series that would be played through cell phones; cell phone technology at the time was more advanced than in the U.S. - we were still catching up.

He bought me a ticket to London and put me up in a tony West End hotel. Chuck is a forward thinker, as it turned out, his idea for a *webisode* series was a few years ahead of its time; no one seemed to have a clue as to what we were talking about, and I felt I'd wasted my friend's time and money by making the trip.

Then I met Chuck's friend "Robert" from Oxford. Robert has a classic professor demeanor, steeped in Eastern mystical thought, a world renowned author and painter who lives between Nepal and London. Shaking his hand, I had the profound feeling *he* was the reason I was in London; Robert shared stories of his travels to Nepal and Tibet, and I wound up spreading some of Luana's previously mentioned ashes behind his home overlooking the Thames River.

Over the next year, I continued my conversation with Robert, his keen mind wrestling with Eastern philosophical concepts, his email missives filled with great bits and pieces of his life. Then one day, I got some horrible news from him - his beautiful daughter Carrina had suddenly passed away in an accident. Robert was devastated. His email contained easily the saddest words I've ever read, but one concept startled me; he said the day of her passing was a day he felt he'd feared his whole life. As he drove to recover her body, he wrote that it felt as if he was replaying an incident he always knew would come.

I'd just read Carol Bowman's "Children's Past Lives" and books by various psychics - James Van Praagh's "Talking to Heaven" for one - and they spoke of reincarnation in a way that seemed to give solace, so I put a list together of some books I thought might help. Robert put together his own list of books for me which included Michael Newton's "Journey of Souls." I opened the book and saw Newton had clients who spoke of being in classrooms "dressed in white" in their life between lives, descriptions of where we go after we die, just as Luana had described, and I decided I'd begin a documentary on the topic.

Robert later told me he'd visited a reputable psychic for help in contacting his daughter, but was unable to do so. The following is an excerpt of his session with a Newton trained therapist in London.

---

[76] "Tibetan Refugee" and "Journey into Tibet" with Robert Thurman

A LIFE IN BOSTON
Robert and *Christine*

(Christine begins the session by taking him back through his life and into a previous one.)

Christine: Describe this past life.
Robert: I'm an adult, male. It's 1842, Boston harbor; there's a clipper ship, I can hear seagulls. It's bright, warm, I'm 36 or 38, wearing a suit made of silk, tight trousers, black shoes, a hat, maybe a cane. I have dark hair, elegant. I'm waiting for someone. My name is Matthew Portland or Pollard.[77] There's my wife, Elizabeth, who is wearing an orangey-red, russet dress with a bustle at the back. She's 32, is sweet, has red/blonde hair, and is tall and elegant.

I feel like there's a colonial house with trees behind and an expanse of grass. It looks Dickensian, with coaches and horses. I'm here with Elizabeth. There's a knowing, a respect and trust - I feel good with her. We're prosperous; we live a rich, full life. It's a warm summer day, there's a breeze blowing through the trees, which have elongated leaves with serrated edges. People are out promenading, there are children around, and it's a park, a nice day out. I have quite a deep voice in this life, I'm quite dapper! I'm tall and straight with dark hair, she has red hair. I work and she does embroidery at home. It's a respectable life. I'm a merchant or work in a bank. It's Boston, somewhere inland.

NOTE: Robert told me he's never been to Boston, but always felt that he'd lived there before.

We're inside. The windows have small panels of around 6"x 8." It's thick Victorian glass, which distorts the view of the street outside. It's bright outside, but there's not much light getting into the room. There's a wall with a big dresser displaying plates, jugs and fine pieces of pottery, decorative rather than useful. The room also has bookshelves and a rocking chair. I can hear a cuckoo clock.

In the next scene I see, Elizabeth is dead. I'm not much older. There is a lot of pain in this life. I know what pain is for – losing what you love.

Go to the last day of this life. Be there now.
I'm sitting at a table by myself, drinking whiskey to drown my sorrows. I have a square decanter and a glass, I'm miserable. I'm 57; I have all my hair, but it's grey. I'm wearing what looks like a military uniform, red and cream regalia. I don't want to live. I can rise above it and see I'm lying on a bed. I've died on my own. I'm above my body, about seven feet above. I can see a light; I'm looking back at my body.

---

[77] Pollard was a common name in Massachusetts in the 1800's. I found a Matthew Pollard in the Massachusetts census records in 1860.

A JOURNEY INTO DEEP SPACE

And after that?

I'm moving slowly, being drawn away. I see amorphous things around me. Splotches of light and color and dark. I feel like I still have a body. I'm looking up, there's a moment of... almost like breathing in the stillness. It's very, very peaceful and still.

There's a strong sensation in my right hand. My hands are dissolving... I'm no longer in physical form. It's energy, a strong energetic form. I'm somewhere in the twilight zone, possibly because of the heavy energy. It's grey, but there's a sense of an enormous sunrise somewhere in front, sun behind clouds. It's the source of energy. It's very strong. I can soak it in.

I'm aware of a deepening that happens, and then I move back into conventional awareness. I can see a nebula; a spiral galaxy, a sun behind clouds. It's a star light, pure white, with countless needle-like rays. The galaxy has huge gaseous clouds, where things are being born. I'm moving towards the galaxy, being drawn, like a kite. There's no fear. It's like I'm learning to be disembodied again.

I feel a presence of beautiful love. It's above and in front; a very loving presence. I feel the presence of... my soul mate. It's wonderful to make this connection. It's almost too much to bear. I could die for love like this. It's a two-way connection, heart to heart. It's angelic, radiant, like a Wesleyan angel with big shoulders, a big form with white rays of light. The love is so strong. The heart of the galaxy is beating with this love; it's the soul of the universe with which we seek to merge. It's sometimes hard for people to understand that capacity for love.

What does your soul do for pleasure?

I hear the music of the universe; incredible music. I go to other places, too. It's like a sci-fi film; I see myself in a place that's yellow and blue, like a desert, with intense deep turquoise. You fly there for the sense of relationship to an environment; it's like a film of the Himalayas taken from a helicopter. Flying on a paean of joy, like a dart from a crossbow. There are other worlds too, atmospheric, multicolored – the colors and contours change. It's exhilarating, fun. I go there alone or with others, flying at a huge velocity. The movement is like a flying saucer, a complete freedom of movement.

The place we arrive at is known as "Sammah." It has volcanic craters, no life. There's another world too, like Mars, silent and red; I'm on the ground here. The sky is golden orange. Then, there's space again, and like a giant skating rink, a planet, "Kieron" or "Kieros;" again, no life. On Sammah it's almost like flying through liquid, like a crystal swan in the sky of suns. Beautiful.

My work in the spirit world is to inspire, to give hope. We need to experience suffering to do this work. I learned that from my sister who died. She was deformed when she was alive; I was 14 when I saw her in spirit form, after she died. She came to me in a vision, and we were flying together through a beautiful sky. In the vision, she was perfect, with no deformity in spirit. She was my first teacher about being able to fly in the spirit world. That experience led me into my work, my studies. I wanted to know what happened, and why? I had to find the answers.

THE COUNCIL OF ELDERS

Let's go to a place of learning.
There are beings here. I have humility and bow before them. They are Elders. They're luminous, white, wearing robes with folds, a little bit like choir boys' robes, pleated. They're radiant white. They wear silver medallions and there are 5 or maybe 6 beings. They're androgynous, but appear as male; in essence, they are who we are, projections of ourselves, our own potentiality. The image I see is like "The Last Supper." They're in a semi-circle, behind a curved panel, a blue light behind. It's a bit like a Sunday school! It's a dome structure made of panels of blue. The curve of the rostrum follows the curve of the dome. The dome is blue, like stained glass within a gold lattice of triangles.

NOTE: Seeing the council of elders wearing medallions is covered in Michael Newton's "Destiny of Souls." Robert had not read his book prior to this session. People say that each medallion represents some insight, or victory they've accomplished during a lifetime.

As I look around, I see there are fine rays of light, and the beings have auras like deities have. I can smell roses and jasmine on my hands, the smell of divinity, of sanctity. It's a cathedral of light with Guides, beings, friends.

My daughter Carrina is my main Guide. Her face is radiant with light… They're like icons; they're not in a complete state. I feel overwhelming awe with these presences… too wise and too enlightened to be human. But it's wonderful.

Let's ask for help in healing the sadness we touched on in your current life.
It's very healing to have these images of seeing Carrina so joyful and not to have the pain of missing her. She's advanced, but advancement on this level… I'm looking into the philosophy rather than any dogma. She can take human form and will again. My work in this world is to take the dogma out and see from our own experience what will help. Human birth is precious, but I believe we have complete freedom to assume any form. Our Guides are us; we are not separate. We have this incredible capacity to assume responsibility rather than place it on our Guides and Elders, although they embody what we aspire to. I would like to take away from this the ability to help people with bereavement.

Put that message to the Elders.
They say, "You do the best you can already." To pay attention to every human, that's what I'm good at. I can keep my attention on them and inspire them. "Be content with what you've got," is the message.

THE LIBRARY OF LIFE SELECTION

I'm going to the Library.[78] There are file containers, very large. I say, "I'd like to take this state I'm in, back with me." Carrina says "You know what to do to reach this state." It's almost as if in this life, I have a telescope but have been looking through the wrong end. I have to not jump to conclusions. That channel is open to me; I just need to go into the quiet place more often and meditate to regain this state.

The files in the library are 2 meters high. There are 4 or 5 rows of them, glowing with light from the back. A spectrum of colors. One of the books from the files spontaneously comes out.

NOTE: In other session people refer to this library as the "Place of life selection." It also mirrors descriptions of the "Akashic records" which supposedly contains all the information of every lifetime in existence. Frequently people speak of going here to learn different outcomes of lives they've led, where they're able to see that if they had made a different choice during their life stream, another (more positive) result would occur. This is also a place where people say they are able to examine possible future lives. These are referred to in the next chapter "Golden Light Within."

Ask for help in the Library.
Looking at the pictures in the books is a bit like looking into a doll's house. There are complex geometrics inside. I see an ancient temple, a sandstone pyramid, like Mayan pyramids. I see within the visuals of the book a structure a bit like the Pompidou Centre. Now I see an image of a steam ship, it's very stormy, a paddle boat sailing with big engines.

Ask for some help in deciphering this.
Carrina says "'I don't want to look at books again Dad!" Some are about the past, some about the present and future. I'd like to look at the point where everything is merged into Source and suffering is ended. There's a symbol of a golden sun, like on the Elders' medallions. It's a 3" diameter golden sun, like a Japanese symbol. There is a lot to see in these books. It's being downloaded at high speed and I will have access to it in the future in my subconscious memory. It's as if it's being downloaded into me.

I'm reading my current life book in the Library – I can smell flowers, hyacinths, flowers of death. I am looking into the future. There's a sharp, sweet smell, an incredible scent. (After a pause) I can see... I know when I will die. My breathing will get worse. I will have the energy to do what I need to. Then I will be gone. People really need to see the transitory nature of life. The soul takes residence in the heart. It's a being of light, concentrated, intense light; the human and the soul are together."

---

[78] As previously mentioned, one of the way stations in many LBL is a life selection library.

Robert's journey mirrors others found in Michael Newton's research. For the skeptical, whether Robert was really able to connect to his daughter seems beside the point – one has the profoundly authentic feeling of seeing and connecting with loved ones who are no longer on Earth. One emerges from these sessions *knowing* they've seen their departed loved ones.

For those who've recently lost a loved one, this kind of therapy can be an incredibly healing experience. By taking this journey through hypnosis into his soul world, Robert was able to spend a few hours with his daughter, and experience the concept she's with him all the time.

What's unusual about this story is that I hadn't spoken to our mutual friend Chuck for nearly 20 years when he called me out of the blue, brought me to London, connected me to Robert. Then after the tragic loss of his daughter, Robert sent me information about Michael Newton. If there's synchronicity here, or if our higher selves in the afterlife help events move along here on Earth, I find it interesting to note that Chuck's call inviting me to London came a year before these events occurred; when I shook Robert's hand and felt as if he was the reason I was in London, it completed a complex sequence of events that led me to start my documentary, and ultimately this book. Perhaps what appears to be coincidence may actually be a complex fabric of planned events - like a tapestry – or a 3d chess match - and the weaving of it begins many years before events went in motion. I've grown fond of saying; "There is no such thing as coincidence or something that happens "out of the blue.""

This past fall, I helped Robert arrange an LBL session in NY for his friend Elizabeth, whom he saw playing the role of his wife in his past life regression. According to Robert, during her session she remembered the same past life together that he did. I find this is an unusual confirmation of this work; it's one thing for a person to remember a past life living with someone else – but when two people see *different therapists* in *different cities* on the other side of the world and have the *same past life memory* – for me that's a confirmation that goes beyond coincidence.

Years ago, I visited a friend where Eric Clapton recorded "Tears in Heaven," the song about the tragic loss of his son. Eric had just finished recording the track, I got to hear it and read the lyrics he'd written by hand. I actually picked up the red guitar pick he used to play the soon to become "Song of the Year" Grammy Award winning tune, his name inscribed on it. A friend gave me one of those picks; in light of this research, every time I see it or hear the song, I think; "The answer to your question is "Yes.""

INTERVIEW WITH CHANDA NANCY BERLATSKY

The following is an interview with a Newton Trained hypnotherapist who works in Sedona. Born with a twinkle in her eye and a permanent smile on her face, Chanda Nancy Berlatsky sees people with a number of different religious backgrounds in her practice, but their sessions are remarkably similar.

Rich Martini: How did you come to this work?
Chanda Berlatsky: I learned Transcendental Meditation in 1971. Within weeks of my initiation I had what for me was a cosmic consciousness moment that changed my perception of life. During my meditation, a very bright iridescent light appeared, seemed to move towards me as I moved rapidly towards it. As I merged with the light, the profound silence was astonishing. Then I saw these chainlike links of light that flowed from me and connected me to everyone and everything, and I saw all of creation interconnected.

I understood that as a part of this something we are everything; apart from it, we are nothing. This realization made my heart open with an unfathomable love for all living things. I wanted to stay in this blissful place forever but the intensity was too great. For weeks, I had a silly grin on my face and felt a deep loving connection to everyone and everything. It was as if I was seeing the beauty of the world and all her inhabitants for the first time. Eventually I wanted to share this experience, so I became a spiritual healer. One day a friend sent me a copy of Dr. Newton's "Journey of Souls" and I thought "This is the missing piece, how I can help people experience what I experienced."

Did you have any childhood experiences with ESP?
When I was four I was in bed, and the ceiling suddenly became transparent. I saw three translucent figures hovering above me. They looked down at me with benevolent amusement – as if I had been here many times before. The image that came to mind was one of those old vinyl LP's that has a scratch in it, and repeats over and over. I realized I'd been here many times before and even though I was only four, I was not amused. I didn't tell my parents as it wasn't something talked about. At 22, I attended a prayer circle and I brought up the subject of reincarnation. The minister said "No, we believe in single lives, in resurrection, not reincarnation." But I had this recollection of something more cohesive that brought people from the afterlife together – it made more sense to me.

FROM UTAH TO ARIZONA

What kinds of people typically come to see you in Sedona?
I see clients from all over the country who read Dr. Newton's books and something clicks; "This seems familiar to me." I facilitate regression for religious traditions such as Hinduism, Christianity, Catholicism, Mormonism, Judaism or paganism. A young woman from the Self Realization Foundation was at odds with her community because of her non-traditional beliefs and wanted to know why. In her session, she recalled a life as a man in a Brahmin sect that followed Krishna. In the Life between Life session, she experienced the eternal nature of her soul and at

the Gateway to the spirit realm, Yogananda was there to greet her and she felt an overwhelming sense of love for the energy of this holy man and felt Yogananda's love for her. Afterwards, she was able to return and live in that community and no longer felt resistance to being there.

A man from Montana visited with hopes of reconciling his experience with the Church of Latter Day Saints. This person was gay and struggled with his gayness and after much counseling and chastisement, had to tell them he couldn't be fixed, so he was excommunicated from the Mormon Church. And although he had a partner, he had this unresolved feeling from the loss of friends and family and was interested in having a Life between Life session to understand why he chose his family. What he realized was that after many lifetimes in a conservative religious setting, he had chosen this life which allowed him to move out of it. He also discovered the most contentious church elder was in his soul group. He realized there was nothing the matter with himself, or anything wrong with the community that expelled him; they were both doing exactly what they were supposed to be doing, and he was able to forgive all the people involved in the excommunication. Being gay was just another vehicle to explore self-acceptance, compassion, forgiveness, and non-judgment in this life.

A different reason motivated a Mormon couple to come from Idaho to see me in Sedona. They read Dr. Newton's books and wanted to see what it was about. For both of them, their session confirmed there was something more accepting and loving than what they were being told in the Church. They went through all the usual signposts were very happy to meet their guide and Council of Elders, but later both decided to continue as Mormons; that was their path. However, they now realized there was something broader and wider than the teachings they were being given by the Church.

SOUL MATES

Any unusual past life regressions you can tell us about?
I had a woman who came to me who really wanted to meet her soul mate; she was successful in every part of her life, but there was still this longing, "Where is my soul mate?" When we got to her soul family, I asked "Is there a primary soul mate here?" She said, "There is one, but I can't go to see him, not yet." We went to the body selection room and other places and every step of the way it was, "Now can we meet your soul mate?" "No," came the answer. But as we got ready to come back, she said "Now I can." As she met him she said "As we merge our energies and souls as one, there is the greatest magnitude of love and every pure emotion possible and there is a light that shoots out from the top of our blending energies. Even though we weren't able to incarnate together in this life, this reunion allows us to leave so much of self with the other that it will last a while." This meeting infused her with the strength to go through the rest of her current life knowing it wasn't meant they'd be together in

this life, but they'd be together again in the future.

A PAST LIFE DURING THE HOLOCAUST

Your own LBL – what's the significance of the memory of dying in the Holocaust have for you?

I've had many past life regressions, but I had never seen my most recent one (where I remembered dying in a concentration camp). I don't remember how old I was when "The Diary of Anne Frank" came out; I saw the movie and was deeply and profoundly affected by it. Whenever I heard European police sirens, it would send chills and I'd be struck with fear. I grew up in Portland and wasn't aware of any Jewish kids, but when I moved to LA, the majority of students were. My reaction was "Oh, my people!" Needless to say, they didn't have the same concept of me – with my blond hair, and green eyes. (Laughs) No way. But when I was in high school, I couldn't go into the showers – a tremendous fear of being naked in them. I flunked out of Physical Education because of it. Later, I began to have some suspicions when I heard this concept of past lives, that I had somehow been connected.

WHAT'S THE PURPOSE OF THIS WORK?

Why is a journey like this significant for people?

To date it's the single most important modality I can offer anyone. It gives them a sense of their immortality, of the importance of their life and journey, and it gives a sense of belonging to something greater than themselves. It's not a gifted psychic telling you who you are or what you've been, or going to a "Channeler" to tell you your past and background; it's experiential, the clients become their own channel. After every single client has an LBL, they aren't the same – some part of them has changed in a positive way and it's a resource that remains for them long after their Life between Lives journey is complete."

For me, Chanda's experience with two Mormon families is telling for all religions. One person who'd been outcast, excommunicated for his sexual orientation, and yet under hypnosis, chose to see how he'd chosen this life on purpose, and forgave those from his soul group who he'd asked to help him before coming here. The other couple saw that their religious dogma was not what it claimed to be, yet still returned to the fold because that's the journey they'd chosen for themselves. It would be beneficial for any religious leader to do past life therapy and a between life session; they'd get a profound sense of why they chose this particular life.

According to this research being gay is a deeply spiritual *choice*. We choose different lifestyles to help ourselves progress spiritually; whether hiding in the closet, or waving the rainbow flag high, each choice brings lessons of the spirit. Some choose difficult lives because they're more advanced, on a higher spiritual level, and are able to endure whatever difficulties are thrown their way. But there are those who can't handle the slings and arrows and commit suicide.

According to this research, this may be done to teach the people who harangued them a lesson in love, as when those bullies pass away *they're going to experience the same humiliation they dished out.* Suicide is an incredible loss, and incredible disruption in thousands of souls' plan, as if someone in an intense chess game suddenly wipes clean the board. But because the basic law of the universe is love and compassion, those who do so are harder on themselves for screwing up the elaborate plans they'd originally made, but didn't fulfill. However, since we're given the ability to have thousands of lifetimes, we all get a chance to make up for whatever mistakes we make. The soul does not die, even if the physical body is taken, deliberately or otherwise, we always have the opportunity to correct the mistakes we've made.

I was asked by a former Tibetan monk, "Why would a person choose being born black in Africa with HIV?" I asked, "But which one of those concepts is negative?" Every life is precious; each offers profound lessons, sometimes to help others see the humanity in themselves or compassion for others. "The Tibetan Book of the Dead," describes an amorphous between life experience where we are not conscious, but attracted by karmic conditions to wind up in a future life, either animal or human.

From what I've been able to gather, this treatise appears to be a life between life session recounted by a single Lama;[79] if two monks had the identical experience, then it could be replicated. Newton's research is based on thousands having the same basic experience journeying through the afterlife, and can be replicated.

According to these sessions, karma is not something that follows us involuntarily, rather it's something we choose to pick up in a future life to experience or balance the energy from lives we've previously lived before. Also the research shows the animal realm to be separate from the human realm – animals of the air, sea, and land each have their own reincarnating hierarchy. Apparently, we can visit our pets in the Afterlife, but we aren't able to return as one. But why would we choose to be born under difficult circumstances?

There are two key concepts at play: one is because the person choosing the difficult life is a more experienced or older soul and can handle it. The difficult life is filled with tests and obstacles of the heart that allow us to progress spiritually in greater leaps (as reported here during an LBL session; "We can advance more in going through one tragedy on Earth than 5000 years on some planet with no conflict."

The other is that we choose hard lives out of compassion for others - our sacrifice can help others as well, the Doctor trying to save us, the mother who adopts us, the father who puts us up for adoption - it all is a reflection and variation of the heart - or the great bliss divine energy of the universe where love and

---

[79] Based on discussions with Tibetan translator Peter Alan Roberts, author of "The biographies of Rechungpa." For a concise and insightful commentary, I highly recommend Robert Thurman's translation of the "Tibetan Book of the Dead.".

compassion reside as well. Choosing a tough life can be the ultimate form of compassion for others.

But what about those who choose a boring life? Is every past life memory filled with drama and tragedy?

"I regard the brain as a computer which will stop working when its components fail. There is no heaven or afterlife for broken down computers; that is a fairy story for people afraid of the dark."

- Stephen Hawking

CHAPTER 16
GOLDEN LIGHT WITHIN

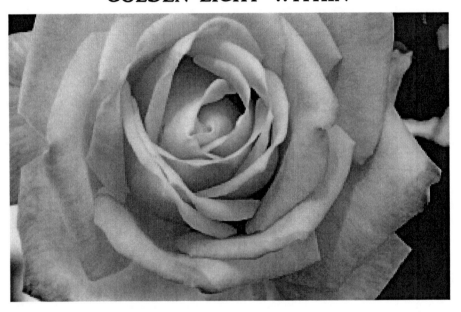

"Love is life. Everything I understand, I understand only because I love. Everything is, everything exists, only because I love. Everything is united by it alone. Love is God, and to die means that I, a particle of love, shall return to the... eternal source."

- Leo Tolstoy

This is an interview with its roots in Russia that I conducted during the Newton Institute conference in Chicago. The session was conducted between two hypnotherapists, one who practices in North Carolina, and the other who is in New York City. Morrin Bass[80] is a striking redhead with an Eastern European accent; this former banker is a hypnotherapist in New York City. *Bryn Blankenship*[81] is a former actress who became a hypnotherapist and moved to North Carolina where she maintains a successful practice.

Bryn: Let's go back to a happy memory in your life…
Morrin: When I was four, laying on the floor in front of the open balcony door in the sunlight, painting a picture with paints, a picture of a tiger. My father was there with me. Teaching me to hold the brush. It feels comfortable and warm.

Let's go back to a time when you were three… Two… One, going back to the time of your birth and going beyond this even, to that very warm, secure place where everything is safe (etc). Let's go to a relevant life… on the count of one, two, and three. Be there now.
It's a carriage, stopping in front of a gate. It's day. It's kind of fall in a city. I'm in front of a large house or palace, there are golden tops of the iron gates and the gates are huge and wide, with elaborate ornaments on them. Beyond is a fountain in front of a big house with many windows. It's where I'm going.

Are you male or female?
I'm a young female, about twenty. Wearing this very tight corset and long, slightly puffy below the waist dress. Lots of lace, the lace is white and the rest of the dress is bluish purple, a very deep color of velvet. I have a matching hat and my hair is made up. I have whitish blond curly hair, and a man helps me out of the carriage with white gloves. I'm with an older man.

What's his relationship to you?
He's bringing me to this gathering, an invitation dinner. It's elaborate; all the lights and people gathering - it's raining and I have a flimsy umbrella. And my shoes are slipping between the gravel pieces.

Describe your shoes to me.
Pointy with a bow. There's a torn spot on the side - I didn't want to wear those.

What's your companion's name?
Vlad. Walesnky. It's 1863 and we're in Russia.
   NOTE: I was able to find a number of Walensky's that were Prussian, as well as Wolinsky, Walinski, and a Countess Walesnki who lived in Moscow in the 1860's. There are references for two Anna Walensky's born in Prussia in the 1830's.

---

[80]   Morrin: New York Awareness Center. www.newyorkawareness.com
[81]   Bryn: www.journeyofsouls.us

A DATE WITH TOLSTOY

What's your companion like?
I feel daughterly submissive, more like he takes care of me. He's very tall, imposing, broad and well-kept man. Black suit, tails, with a cane and a top hat. He has a moustache. He's a banker; I don't work, I just learn. I read, I stay in a small place upstairs and I have lots of books.

What's your interest?
Romantic literature. Novels. My favorite author is something with a T. Toyskay.

Take a deep breath, you'll find the answer comes easily.
Tolstoy.[82] There's something romantic about this style and dress that we don't wear any more. The palace seems so big.

Are you ready to go in? What do you notice?
It's very bright. Everybody's so well dressed and polite. I see my mother. She feels like my mother, but looks younger. (Gasps) I know what this is; my father found me, brought me here and this is where I'm going to live, this is my family, my new home. (Cries) I was lost before. I lived someplace else.

How did you come to be lost?
I came from another mother; my father brought me here to live here with my family. My sister, my older sister and my mother are all greeting me. They call me Anna, or Anichka, the diminutive. My little sister Maria is 13. Very pretty little girl, white dress, pretty curls around her face. She can play piano.

Do you recognize her in your current life?
She's my mother.

How about the other sister? Younger than you?
Her name is Natalia. She has dark hair pulled back with a bow. She's 16.

Do you recognize her in your current life?
She's my aunt. And the man who brought me, who's the father... He feels like my brother in this life. I don't feel close to him. My mother's name is Irina. She feels like my grandmother in this life. She looks like 35, 40, very young.

---

[82] By 1863, Tolstoy had written "The Cossacks" and four other novels. "War and Peace" came two years later.

Why have you all gathered at this event?
Because it's where they live, so they can meet me. It feels like I came from some village, on the periphery, the place where I was raised. I was sponsored by my father, but I had to work. I can sew, I can dance, and I just about got a job with the theater when I came here, so I'm sort of wary because I'm starting to build myself and I kind of like dancing.

Let's move to the next significant event. Tell me what's happening.
I'm in my 40's. I'm in that big house by myself. Sitting in the chair, sewing something.

Are you married?
No, I'm an old maid.

How do you spend your time?
Just helping around the house, my mother. My sisters are all married, even little Maria. I just don't go anyplace.

Was there a significant person in your life previous to this?
Yes and he was killed in the war. He was some army, military something. His name was Alexander Waltensky.[83] He died and I decided not to pursue anything anymore. I have a bluish grayish dress buttoned up to my neck, white lace on top of it. I'm a boring person. God am I boring! Sewing all day, doing house stuff. Ugh. I got disappointed after my fiancée died in the war or something. I feel a lot older than I am, I'm almost dead. Feels like that's how I'm passing the time.

NOTE: One criticism about past life regression is that "Everyone thinks they were Cleopatra." This occurs when a trained therapist isn't available to ask the probing questions about the details of a remembered past. More importantly, the question of why a person chose a particular past life, and the connection of why they chose this one is left unexamined. Morrin eventually comes to the reason why it was important for her to remember this "boring" existence.

Was there more life to you before Alexander died?
I was very hopeful, to be with him, to have a family. His death changed all that. He was a military officer and traveled a lot. I stayed in the house, felt very devoted. I guess I stayed devoted. I see there's a stack of letters, with blue ribbon tying them together, which I carefully keep behind the piano in a little wooden box. I play the piano often. What a boring life! (Cries) Just sadness over this life.

I want you to move forward to the next significant event... one... Two... Three...
My father dies and I'm by myself now. I'm 53. I'm joyful; I'm getting rid of the house. I am in the carriage moving to the country. There's a rose garden and a small little cottage. There's an old woman there, happy old woman.

---

[83] Felix and Paulina Waltenskj emigrated from Russia to the U.S. in 1903

Who is she?
She's my nanny where I grew up. I call her "Nana." It's a village near the river.

How did you come to live with the Walesnkys?
My mother was connected to my father, but wasn't married. She wasn't from a good family. But he was in love with her and she died. She was very sick; I was three when she died. I lived in the little cottage and then moved closer to the city to find work, when my nanny wrote a letter to my father, in the hopes he would help. That's when he found me.

What happens next?
The next is... I die.

Go ahead to the time of death, but moments before.
I got attacked on the road when I walked to the village. I was 61.

How many attackers?
Two men put a knife into my stomach and took my purse and left me there lying on the side of the road - they pulled me behind the bushes.

Let's move from there and look at this from a detached sort of way. Do you stay with the body?
I stayed with it for a few days, hovering until I was found. I just don't care about the funeral.

NOTE: It's common for a person who's been killed in some manner to stay around until the body is buried or found. According to this research, people are outside of time when they're outside of their bodies, so staying around a particular location isn't a matter of time, but emotion. They may feel the need to stick around further for some reason, no matter how long it is; hence the reports of "haunted castles" or houses for centuries. When the spirit feels they've spent enough time in remorse, or reminiscing, their spirit guide reportedly shows up and suggests it's time for the soul to return home, or head "into the light." Since free will rules the Universe, it's up to the soul to decide when to go there.

A CONTEMPLATIVE LIFE

What did you learn from this life?
It was an emotionally restful life to contemplate on purpose. To stay in touch with the Earthly reality and prepare myself for the more involved life (I have now). And also to let go. I just couldn't let go. I stopped every activity I wanted to do, every emotion I wanted to feel. I stopped myself from moving ahead. I tucked in my identity, didn't become who I wanted to be, or needed to be.

Was anything left uncompleted?
All of my relationships, my love, my profession; uncompleted.

What made you the happiest in this life?
I thought I'd be happy living in that big house with the rest of the family who wasn't my family. With all the glitter. But I wasn't.

So how was it for you all those years in that house? Did you blend with the family?
No. It was so flat and gray and boring. In the end I didn't know how old I was. It feels like the first time I felt joy was when I moved away from that house.

How does this relate to your life now?
In that life it was a physical and emotional preparation, and a mental preparation, because I didn't do very much, or feel very much at all. I didn't explore myself.

And what do you do now in your current life?
I'm exploring and doing and learning. I didn't feel love in that life - I felt welcomed, but I didn't feel love. It was a sad place.

NOTE: The hypnotherapist began the session asking for the person to view a previous existence that has some effect on the current one. As we'll see in a few moments, despite her remembering this life as a boring one, there were spiritual lessons learned.

THE JOURNEY BACK

Allow your spirit to move to a healing place.
I see purple and blue just streaming through me and the outline of that light is just golden light and it streams right through me out of nowhere, through the top as if I'm dissolved and I don't have a body. It's just the stream of energy that is washing away and I'm embracing it with my essence since I don't have a body. But at the same time it feels like I'm floating upward through that light - that's a familiar feeling. I float upward to meet it from wherever it comes from, float up there and let it flow through me endlessly. It's bright, golden light with white inside; it's purple on the outside.

Allow yourself to feel that.
There's somebody waiting.

When this is complete, we'll speak to that person. Let me know when it's complete.
It's like a waterfall. It's like an infusion and waterfall. He's taken me by the arm and pulled me outside the waterfall and said "Are you ready now?"

Who pulled you out?
He's my guide. I didn't even recognize him. Michael. He has a white outline as if he's a white light cutout. Little round on top as if there's a head with long hair, but I can't see any details, it's just blinding white light. So loving and inviting.

And what message does he have for you today?
He says "You're an emotional soul, you like to worry, but there's nothing to worry about." He says "You have a big life coming up." (She cries) So it was helpful to rest a little.

That's wonderful.
(Cries) I'm trying to find what emotion this is. There's no word for it. A cross between joy and love, there's no particular object for me to look at to experience this emotion, but it's so strong.

What if we ask Michael for an object to hold in your mind that will remind you?
He says. "You want an object? Here it is." He gives me a big red heart cut out, like a paper heart. He says "You can place it inside your heart." When I turned to place it inside my heart there is like a ball of energy, light. There's no room to put it in. He takes me as if by the hand, and says "Come, I'll show you something." And it's like as if in the blackness of the cosmos with stars all over the place there's a place with green grass and a bench. And there we are sitting down, like people.

Like people?
Like people would sit on a bench, as if we were people. He says "Rest your eyes on this lovely scenery, there are flowers in the sunshine, sunset, and the green grass and the trees." And there's some people - so you don't feel lonely, this place is occupied. I feel as if I'm a ball of light and at the same time, a person. "What is this place?" and he says "This is where we decide what you're going to do next."

NOTE: This is a common occurrence during a life between life session, where the client is taken to the library or place where they're able to choose their next incarnation. Sometimes people describe being able to view a physical book that has moving images within it that depict the life to come, they also report that they're able to test out those lifetimes briefly, as if they were diving into the book and getting a brief glimpse of a possible life. There are also depictions of viewing future life possibilities in a 3 dimensional way, as if on movie screens, but they're completely interactive. Usually a guide of some sort escorts them and helps them to sort out who and what they want to be.

THE LIFETIME LIBRARY

And what kinds of things is he showing that you'll be doing next?
It's as if he's showing me where I could go next. There are different scenes – from

left to right - on the left there is a city, in the middle there's a mountain scene, like a Tibetan mountain, something snowy on top. And then there's another nature scene, to the right of that with a lot of snow -- I don't want to go there! Snow is not for me. (Laughs) "Choose your environment first," he says, "and you'll get a task to do there." So I choose the city on the left.

What city is that?
Paris. It's not a contemporary scene either.

What year?
1900's. Beginning of the 20th century. He says "Wait a minute I'm going to show you something else." Ah.

SOUL MATE

My beloved. My fiancée from my previous life. He comes out in uniform so I recognize him.

Is he in your current life?
He takes the uniform off and says "I don't need that disguise anymore." His light is nice. He has a soft, turquoise light, a little bit of orange on the outside. That's a pretty combination. His light is very loving. He is my current partner in this life.
NOTE: Morrin realizes that her soul mate had been in the previous life – that he was the soldier who she'd fallen in love with, and that he has been with her for many lifetimes, including her current one.

THE GLOWING LIGHT WITHIN

Take a moment with your guide.
There's this very bright light everywhere I look; I'm part of it. He's showing me I'm part of a universal plan, I'm part of that light and it's everywhere, there's nowhere in the universe there isn't this light. He says "That's what you're working with, keep it as part of you and bring it back." We need to know there's nothing else but light and love. The work we're doing (as hypnotherapists) is about light, because it opens us up to understanding. We're on a mission to clarify and create more light and love and it's available to everyone; all we have to do is open ourselves to it. The light is clear and cleansing, loving and peaceful. Eventually when we become light all the other things go; sadness and such. It's very healing.

It doesn't really matter where you are.
My guide is saying "It really doesn't matter in the end what you do, you just have to do what you choose with the light."
In Morrin's session, she recalled an "incredibly boring" life, proving not every past life is iconic, dramatic or even memorable. She lived in fear of life, and wound

up as an old maid, waiting for her lover to return from war. But while examining her life between lives, she was able to reconnect to her soul mate, this man who was her fiancée in a previous life and is now in her current life.

But what are "soul mates?" People report everyone has a soul group of usually 3-25 different people who travel through their various lives. There is often a primary soul mate, someone who plays a role of significance in a lifetime, unless, as in Morrin's previous life, they agree in advance not to do so.

I began to query people and found nearly everyone can exactly pinpoint the moment they met their future wife or husband in great detail. People under hypnosis claim these events are planned in advance, and the actual meeting is like a déjà vu memory of a meeting preplanned between lives. The veil of forgetfulness lifts for a moment, and two souls reconnect.

I was struck by her imagery of the 'glowing light' that emanated from within. I had a similar experience one afternoon, while sleeping, I suddenly felt myself dissolve into a sea of atoms of golden light. I felt connected to everything in the Universe. I was outside of time, and could visit any point on the timeline at will, but especially where a photograph of me existed, as if the photo was a slice of time. It was the most blissful moment I'd ever experienced before I passed out.

But the interviews and research were showing that we are fully conscious between lives, even if we experience a blissful dissolution into energy. And that while fully conscious we choose our next lifetime. People choosing their parents? I began to wonder about my own children; had my wife and I chosen them, or had they chosen us?

"I am in exact accord with the belief of Thomas Edison that spirit is immortal, that there is a continuing center of character in each personality. But I don't know what spirit is, nor matter either. I suspect they are forms of the same thing. I never could see anything in this reputed antagonism between spirit and matter. To me this is the most beautiful, the most satisfactory from a scientific standpoint, the most logical theory of life."

- Henry Ford

CHAPTER 17
MY SON THE MONK

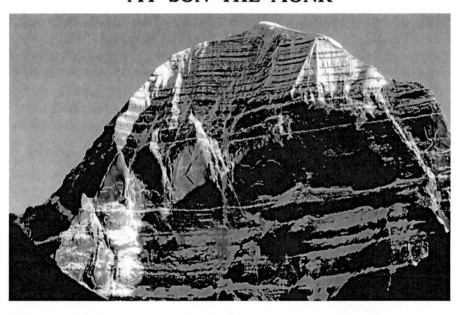

"Often the child has quite precise details. If one accepts the possibility of reincarnation, one can entertain the idea that children demonstrate skills, even genius that are logical results of previous experiences."

- Dr. Ian Stevenson

Robert Thurman told a story about his daughter Uma that points to how people may be aware of their life's destiny, but not conscious of it. After leaving the Tibetan monkhood, Robert returned with his wife Nena to Dharamsala where he studied with the famous Dr. Donden, the Dalai Lama's physician. And at some point, Bob was hired by Amherst College in Massachusetts, so he gathered up his family and they trekked to New England. By this time Uma was a toddler and had little exposure to western culture. One day the family went to purchase clothes for the cold New England winter; based on a professor's salary, they made use of a local thrift shop. At some point, young Uma disappeared, and the family was frantic. Then, they finally found her in a clothing store; she was dolled up in a fancy cowboy outfit complete with red hat and boots.

Her dad tried to explain that on a professor's salary, they wouldn't be able to afford the fancy duds. She replied, "It's okay daddy, when I grow up I'm going to be a big movie star and will be able to afford all the clothes I want."

I met Professor Thurman in an unusual way. Just after Luana passed, I took a job working for our mutual friend Charles Grodin on his talk show on CNBC. Charles had helped his friend through her long illness, and he offered me a job on his award winning talk show. On the plane to NY, I happened upon an article about Robert Thurman, who was the first Westerner ordained by the Dalai Lama as a monk in the Tibetan Buddhist tradition. Robert wrote about the day he'd met his reincarnated master, the teacher who'd overseen his education before he left the monkhood. He'd gone to the reincarnated tulku's home in Dharamsala, India, not far from where the Dalai Lama lives for an unannounced visit. After he knocked on the door, Robert was led to a patio where the five year old boy was riding his tricycle.

At some point he saw Thurman and rode over and stopped at his feet. Robert says he squinched his face up at him and said "Thurman, why did you leave the monkhood? You made me so disappointed!" Robert said the boy's face at that moment resembled his former teacher's, and Robert found himself fumbling through an answer about how becoming a teacher at Columbia University allowed him to spread the dharma of Buddhism. The child seemed satisfied with his reply, and went back to riding his trike.

As I read that story, I thought, "Well, if there's anyone on the planet who might know how I can get in touch with my departed friend Luana in the afterlife, it would be Robert." When I got to my desk at CNBC, I called and asked him if I could audit his class. He warned me that it was an advanced philosophy requirement for doctoral candidates only; "How familiar are you with Hegel and Kant?" he asked. "They play for the 49ers" I said. He chuckled and allowed me to sit in for the twelve week session.

Sitting in his classroom is like surfing a meteor shower trying to capture complex concepts hurtling past you at light speed. The ideas and concepts so facile, complex, I felt like someone in the parking lot outside the ballpark. I'd have to re-read passages of Thurman's textbook "Fundamental Guide To the Middle Way" just to make sure they were in English. But I became enamored of Robert and his insight, and when the opportunity arose to go to India with him, I jumped at the chance. Later, I offered my services to film a documentary of his next trip to Tibet, and while I was melting from the heat in a sound stage in New Delhi, making a Bollywood movie I'd written called "My Bollywood Bride," an email arrived inviting me to Katmandu, where'd I'd join Bob and a group of 25 tourists making their way across Tibet and to do a circumnavigation of the famed Mt. Kailash, considered by the Hindus, Buddhists, Bon and Jain religions to be the "Center of the Universe." How could I pass it up?

As I traveled with Robert around India and Tibet, he gave talks and meditations in various parts of the "Land of the Snows," and would lecture on a variety of topics, including life and death, and the Tibetan book of the dead, which he'd done a masterful translation of. He'd give guided meditations about the "Jewel Tree" myth of Tibet, and taught me how to formally meditate. Traveling with him I got a chance to learn about India, Nepal and Tibet first hand, and their peerless philosophy. I also got a chance to learn more about the Buddhist concept of reincarnation, and how it works with realized masters.

Sometime later, I was in Chicago visiting my mother when my wife Sherry put my two year old son on the phone. We'd said a few words together in his wee vocabulary - mostly, "I love you," or "I miss you." So fully expecting him to say something of the sort, I was shocked when he said "Dad, I was a monk in Nepal!" I paused for a few seconds. Did he just say what I thought he said? "Put your mom on the phone, honey." Sherry confirmed she'd heard him say it, but had no idea why he said it. He'd said it as if he'd been waiting for two years to say that sentence, and could finally formulate it.

When Sherry was pregnant, a friend said she dreamt that the friend was standing on a bus stop, and a pregnant Sherry had said "I'm going to have a baby in Nepal." This friend didn't know that Sherry was pregnant, and no, Sherry's never been to Nepal, and rarely outside her native Utah.

When my son RJ was born, Sherry had him resting on her chest while he was sleeping. She had a profound vision of white mountains and what looked like a monastery. Then she saw a woman in a traditional Tibetan dress, the multi-colored apron they wear that signifies a married woman. She saw two boys in the house, both of them were young monks. She got the feeling that they were the sons of this woman. She said she then got a powerful feeling of sadness from RJ, that he was "missing the solace" of that mountain retreat, wherever it was. But she'd never spoken to him of this vision.

I later asked RJ where he was from in Nepal. He said it was "in the mountains." I asked my daughter Olivia, who was 4 at the time, if she remembered RJ "from before." She said "Oh, yes, he was a monk." I hadn't told her what he'd said to me on the phone. "Really?" I said. She said "Yes, he was an old, old monk and everyone came to see him." I asked how she knew him. "I was his doctor," she said. "And when he died, his robes just fell away!" She said that gesturing with her arms open, as if it was a magical experience. Granted, most parents would nod and assume their child was talking about an episode of "Scooby Doo." But he'd already told me he was a monk in Nepal. The words "Rainbow death" entered my head when she made this gesture, and I researched the term.

It's been reported when a highly realized Tibetan lama or monk is about to die, they sometimes enter an equipoise state and are left alone in a room for several days. When the attendants open the doors, the body is gone, and just a robe, with bits of hair and fingernails, remain. It's referred to in the "Tibetan Book of the Dead" as a "rainbow death" because rainbows appear after the disappearance of the monk.

Sometimes as RJ falls asleep, Sherry has observed him open his eyes, stare in the distance, bring his palms together and pray softly to someone only he can see. When asked what he's praying about, he said "To save the Earth. From the people." I assume, or hope, he means from pollution. Either way, both my wife and I have seen him do an elaborate ritual of bowing, turning his hands inside and outward in a "mudra" fashion, (a dance of the hands, that Buddhists say guides energy flow to the brain) which ends with him touching his forehead to the ground and then giggling uncontrollably when he sees we've been watching.

Sherry was having dinner with Olivia and RJ one night while I was away. RJ was three and Olivia five. As they were chewing their pizza, Olivia said quietly to her mom, "I knew your mother before she died; that's how I came to life." Sherry asked her to describe her mother. She did, accurately, hair color, her delight in lounging by the pool of their home in St. George, Utah. Sherry's mother had passed away six years before Olivia was born, so it wasn't clear what she was saying about her death being her entry point to this life. Olivia said "That's how it works. Someone in your family dies so someone new can come into your family." Did she mean "soul group?"

Sherry then asked her, "Did mommy and daddy choose you, or did you choose mommy and daddy?" She said happily, "Oh, I chose you. Daddy was in London and I liked his smile, and you were in an apartment in Venice and you were just... Love." We'd never told her about Sherry's apartment in Venice, nor mentioned my trips to Europe, where I'd stop in London on my way to or from the Cannes Film Festival (the last trip being in 1997, which was about the time of her mom's passing).

One day I had a large picture book from Tibet on the floor. Olivia was flipping the pages, with her little brother RJ looking over her shoulder. She came upon a photograph of the Potala Palace, one of the most famous buildings in the world, where the Dalai Lamas lived in Tibet. It's a massive structure with multiple levels, towers that are painted white, some that are painted red. Olivia pointed to the white towers and said "I used to live up there."

RJ wanted in on the story. He said "I used to live up there too." She said "No, you didn't, you used to live over here..." she pointed to the front of the Potala, across the street, where common people lived in years past. "You lived here because you were from the land of no people, and I was from the land of people." Something about the way she said it rang a bell with me, and I went to the computer to search for the phrase "land of people" and "Tibet." Turns out that's how Tibetans refer to themselves, or at least those folks who hail from Kham, which is known as "The Land of People." Those who aren't from Tibet would be known as being from the "Land of No People," the same way people in Maine consider everyone who wasn't born in Maine to be "from away," whether they're from Vermont, or Sri Lanka.

A few days later, I opened up the book of photos of the Potala Palace and asked RJ if he knew who lived in one of the bedrooms. He shrugged. I asked again. He said "Boba." I looked that up later as well - it's how Tibetans refer to themselves, as in the famous character in Star Wars known as Boba Fett - George Lucas had learned enough about Tibet and some names inhabit his world beyond our world; Boba Phett speaks Tibetan on screen. I'm told "Boba" means "Tibetan" to a Tibetan.

I was driving around Santa Monica with RJ one day when he was three. Sherry and Olivia had stepped out of the car, and I looked at him in the rear view mirror, sitting in his car seat. I said "RJ, do you remember Daddy from before?" He nodded. I said "Where did you meet daddy?" He said simply; "Tibet." My jaw dropped. I said "Where in Tibet?" He said "On the path."

That took my breath away. Did he mean "on the spiritual path?" or did he mean literally on a path? And when did he ever hear the word path? He wasn't in pre-school, and I'd never heard it in any of the myriad Scooby Doos and Sesame Streets he'd seen - and we had no paths near our house. But he clearly said "on the path." I hesitated. I had been on many paths in Tibet while shooting "Journey into Tibet" for Tibet House in New York. Then I remembered something that happened on one particular path in Tibet.

While I was on Mt. Kailash with Robert Thurman in Western Tibet, we came to a point on the path considered particularly sacred; the north face of Mt. Kailash, according to Professor Thurman, is the spot where an individual can make a wish, and it will come true. When he said that, I chuckled to myself, thinking about what my possible wish could be.

I considered two possible choices; money or a film deal. After all, struggling as I have my entire career, it's always a conundrum; which is more important? The work or the money? "A million dollars" or "A Three Picture Deal" - I debated which one to say aloud. I said to myself when I counted down from ten, and got to one, whatever I'm supposed to say would pop out of my mouth.

"Three, two, one…" and out came the words "I want a son."

I was stunned to hear myself say it. It hadn't been part of my conscious mind, my beautiful eight month old daughter was waiting for me back in Los Angeles, and we'd yet to consider having another child, let alone pick a gender.

Which leads us back to the car in Santa Monica, and my son having said he found me "on the path" in Tibet. "Did you find me on Mt. Kailash?" He shook his head, no. I thought about the many dirt paths I'd been on in Tibet, and then remembered my son is very literal. "Was it on Kangra?" I asked. "Yes, Kangra," he said. Kangra is the Tibetan name of the path where I had made the wish. But I'd said the word to him. So I couldn't really be sure if that's what he meant.

While I was on the film "Salt," I sublet an apartment in the West Village. While I was on set one day, RJ found some books in the sublet sitting next to a small table. He threw one into the trash. My wife said "What are you doing?" "That book is worthless," he said. "This is the important one." He held up Robert Thurman's "Circling the Sacred Mountain," about Robert's first trip to Tibet. Sherry says RJ opened the book to a picture of the North Face of Mt. Kailash, (where I made the wish) and said "*That's where I found Daddy.*"

Wow.

Past life and life between life research shows the same startling revelation; we choose our parents, we choose our lives – sometimes to help our parents, siblings or friends through some kind of a crisis, sometimes because the life we choose will allow us to progress spiritually to a place which will help us fulfill our destiny.

Recently the New York Times published an article about how interest in reincarnation is increasing.[84] Dr. Weiss, the Yale trained psychiatrist, best-selling author, has been holding classes in past life regression. Dr. Weiss is quoted as saying "Any good therapist can use these techniques, and you can learn them in a week." However, the difference between most past life regressionists and Michael Newton trained ones is the ability to take a client between lives and examine why they chose a past life, and why they chose this one, and the connection between the two, and how highlights in our lives may be preplanned.

When people meet those who'll have a profound influence on their life, especially lovers or soul mates, they frequently have the feeling "I knew I was going to be with this person." I've interviewed couples who claim the moment they met their soul mate in this life, they knew they'd marry (including a friend who met her husband when she was 8 and knew they'd marry 20 years later.) A friend saw her future husband interviewed on a program and "Knew he was the man I'd marry" as if the message was in past tense. I spoke to a young New York newlywed who said that his in-laws had a similar amazing story. When his wife's mother was 11 years old, she fell into a pond in a park in Brooklyn. A young boy came over and

[84] "Interest In Reincarnation is Growing," by Lisa Miller. NY Times 8-29-2010

fished her out of the mud. As the unknown boy walked away, she turned to her friend and said "That's the boy I'm going to marry." And they did.

When I was in USC film school in the early 80's, I met a tall blond actress on campus and asked if she'd appear in my student film. She was taking acting classes at the University and was interested in pursuing a career in film, so the 18 year old ingénue said yes. One day while chatting with her between classes she said "I'm going to marry Jackson Browne." I asked if she'd ever met him. She said "No, but I just know that I'm going to be with him one day." The actress was Daryl Hannah, and in 1980's, they spent nearly a decade together.

While I was researching a film script, I met Tom Tureen, an attorney in Maine who'd met his wife in a Church in New York. One night while walking in the city, Tom was drawn into a chapel where he heard a choir singing. He looked at a girl in the front row and knew she was going to be his wife. It took him months to track her down, and then appeared unannounced at her college dorm. He told her his saga, and as they spoke, a meteor streaked across the sky. He claimed it was a sign from heaven they were meant to be together. And so they've been ever since.

Even Bruce Springsteen and Clarence Clemons described their first meeting as something magical. Clemons claimed he felt compelled to see Bruce's band the night he took his saxophone to a club. Springsteen claims a bolt of thunder cracked overhead during a storm; when the door to the club opened, lightning revealed the saxophonist standing in the doorway. He came onstage and played, and the rest is musical kismet and a 40 year history between two great musicians.

In the interview with Michael Newton, he describes in detail how he'd spent his life trying to find a "nurse named Peggy," and in her interview, Peggy recounts the day that he found her – they've never been apart since.

In my case, I spoke to my wife for about a half an hour before I said casually (startling myself) "Why don't we just get married and have a couple of kids?" (She now claims I say that to everyone I meet at Starbucks. Ba-dum-bum.)

As mentioned, while filming "Salt," I was chatting with the actor who plays the President in the film, Hunt Block. Somehow the conversation spun around to past lives, and a New York Police Detective, who was working on the film as an advisor, overheard our conversation. He pulled me aside and said "What do you know about reincarnation?" in a way that only a New York Cop could ask the question, like my life depended on the answer. I told him I was working on a documentary and only knew what people had told me. "Well my daughter has a problem," he said. "She claims she lived in Australia. And we've never been there." He also said that since she was a little girl, she claimed to see "A man in uniform," standing in the kitchen from time to time.

The Detective couldn't figure out who she might be talking about, until he discovered a wallet photo of his former partner, who'd died years ago. "Who is this?" he asked his daughter. She smiled. "That's the man I see in the kitchen

Daddy. He wears a uniform just like you." The Detective wanted to know if one story could be connected to the other. I told him I'm no expert, but from what I've learned, they could be; I'm told children under seven generally have a better ability to remember past lives, or see people no longer on the planet than the rest of us do.

He said, "So what do I do about this past life stuff? It's bothering her." I said "Well, take out a map of Australia and see what she says. If she's making it up, the details will be all over the place, if she's remembering it, it'll be consistent." The next day he excitedly pulled me into a back room to share his news. "I did what you said, I took out the map, and she pointed to a town called Perth and said "That's where I lived with my family, daddy! They were farmers, and I died in a drought there!" He said he did his best to not be shocked by the information, and let her express, and come to terms with her feelings about the memory.

An ad came on the television with a beautiful young model wearing a skimpy bra and angel wings. She was dancing provocatively, selling the latest in lingerie. My 3 year old son stood up and pointed excitedly at the set. "Daddy!" he said, staring at the model and then looking at me. "I want that!" I chuckled, knowing he'd told me he remembered being a monk in a past life. "But RJ," I protested, "I thought you were a monk." "Not anymore!" he said happily.

My son claimed he found me in Tibet. My daughter claimed she found my wife in Venice, California and me in London – both places we'd never told her we'd been. Under hypnosis, people were saying they chose their future lives; they chose their parents. That's a mind bending, life altering proposition.

People claimed under hypnosis that they didn't always reincarnate on Earth – that there were other planets, or planes that they spent time visiting. Some people even claimed that they normally didn't reincarnate here on Earth, and that it was an anomaly that they had this time around. I was surprised to actually find one.

"Reality is merely an illusion, albeit a very persistent one."

- Albert Einstein

CHAPTER 18
OVER THE RAINBOW

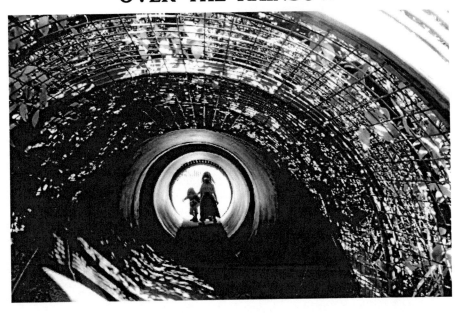

"Everyone's quick to blame the alien."

- Aeschylus

There's no place like home.
After having filmed a number of Scott De Tamble's hypnotherapy sessions, I mentioned if there were any sessions he had that were out of the ordinary, to ask the client if it would be all right for me to use it. A few weeks later, three hour session on CD came to me in the mail with the note "Hey Rich, check this out - pretty interesting."

I transcribed the session for Scott and his patient, whom I'll call Thomas. Thomas had read some of Michael Newton's books, and found Scott listed on the website. Since he didn't live far away, he felt it was kismet for him to see Scott. He felt he'd been suffering his entire life from "being in the wrong body." This can take the form of behavioral issues, it can result in suicidal thoughts; with the help of a trained hypnotherapist, some are able to sort out why they have these feelings. However, a bit more was uncovered in the following session:

Scott De Tamble & Thomas

Scott: Before birth, and inside the womb, inside your mother now, feel the protection of this dark warm environment, all around you... feeling safe and protected.
Thomas: I'm not in the womb.

What's happening?
(Deep sigh). I decided to come here very quickly, because I needed to. I've got things to do with these folks; I need to be with these people. So I missed all that (gestation) - that's what some of my sadness is from, (missing) that bonding that comes biologically. I accepted the templates as is.

Tell me more. Breathe and talk to me about this experience.
I really can't remember anything younger than maybe 3 or 4 years old - I can remember being in the kitchen in one of our earliest houses. I think I'm 3 or 4.

Tell me about this template thing. You accepted the templates "as is?"
I wanted to be in this body and I was part of (the planning of) it, part of the desire (to be here), it wasn't all my desire, it was also the other beings desire, and we agreed to do this. I don't know who that other being is (who helped plan this life), maybe we'll find out. But I have a great body, a great family.

So this other being needed the womb and birthing process and earlier life?
That's all they needed. We transferred. Okay, this is going to sound really weird, but there's a spaceship out there that brought me here.

NOTE: This is very uncommon, and Newton says the research shows that there are no "drop-ins" to a person's life trajectory. Scott repeatedly came back to explore this concept to see if perhaps he was confusing it in some manner. Thomas claimed his spirit guide had taken his place for the first few years of his current life, something unheard of in the research. Scott is trained in revisiting story points later on during a session to see if a patient might have a different insight later on. He's also trained to not doubt a story, rather to ask a series of questions that allow the patient to delve deeper, even if a spaceship is involved.

BROTHER FROM ANOTHER PLANET

Tell me about it.
I don't want to tell you about it.

What do you mean "There's a spaceship?"
It's a place that I go on occasion, I call it a dream, but I go there.

What do you do on this ship?
I'm working on something. I come back to this place all the time because I love it so much.

This place?
Yes, Earth. I've been here so much, it's a project, but it's not my home.

So you love the Earth, it's like a project and you spend a lot of time here?
Yes, I'm here a lot. There's a lot of home-like stuff about it, but it's not home.

Why does this bring sadness to you?
Just *this life*. I missed out on some really important transference on the soul level because I didn't choose to come through during the gestation period - I knew that was going to be a liability, but there would be beings and opportunities to help correct it - you're one of them, Scott - thank you, it's nice to see you, today; it's been a long wait.

It's my pleasure and my honor. Tell me about...
We're getting ready to move to another species altogether, it's happening on a DNA level.

Who's getting ready to move?
This planet.

To another planet?
No, the human species, of which you and I are part.

A PLANETARY JUMP IN CONSCIOUSNESS

We're poised to make a huge jump in consciousness and it's happening already among us. I'm just one of the workers working on that; it's been a pet project for a long time.

So tell me about this jump.

It's a shift in our DNA, awakening parts of our apparatus that have been closed down - when we come into these bodies; we shut down much of our awareness and our abilities to be encapsulated. And yet there's much in these bodies we can draw upon and be open to. As a species, we're evolving and it takes little interventions, and many people working on many levels to make that happen. There are many light-beings here - even if they're not aware that they're aware; they're aware. I'm one of those.

And what is your work exactly?

It's opening the heart to all the diversity, to all the beauty. To feel the pain, transport the pain, let it be, so it can be set free. Being a light-being and animal, we've had so much strife in our 'animalness' struggling back and forth. Yet we're driven by it, and we can't help it. Only when we tune into our higher self can we let the animal be and it's no longer driven with out-of-control passions.

Why do we use these animal bodies, then?

Because it's a glorious expression of "all that is"... one of the glorious expressions. We bring great joy to "all that is." It's a lot of work, but it's also a lot of fun.

So this is sort of work and sort of an adventure for you being on this project.

Yes, it *is* an adventure.

"Project Earth." What's the home place? Where do the space ships come from?

(After a pause) This is what I'm waking up to today; it's been knocking on my door for quite a while, but only seriously the past year... The ships come and go to relieve us; it's not a 'leaving of the body and going back to the spirit realm,' it's disengagement from the physical for a span of time and getting a recharge and then coming right back to doing what we're doing.

What's the process?

I'll recount the last one I remember. I was teleported into a room with no boundaries, it was milky white; there were beings all around me, feathering me with their long graceful hands. They're loving and they're warm and comforting and I'm feeling very at peace, and the movement then becomes more intense, and more attentive with an intention behind it; I'm being touched on the inside, I can feel things molecularly inside my being that are being rearranged. I had this done previously, as I remember it was really, really intense and when they sensed my alarm, they offered soothing thoughts, and it helped a little bit. But they knew it wasn't going to help a lot - they just had to do what they had to do. I knew it was going to be intense so they just did it as fast as possible; tied knots, pulled cords, loosened strings, threw me back down and I got up.

NOTE: For anyone who's read about "alien abduction" this is a common theme – taken aboard a ship and touched, accompanied by telepathic thoughts of comfort. (Not everyone is comforted) However this is the first I've heard of an alien abducting "one of their own," to help make adjustments.

When was this?
Feb 18th, 2002.

How were you altered or changed from that treatment?
On a physical level, it increased my spirit energy dramatically, it revved my immune system, it realigned imbalances, it was a profound effect that with time began to manifest. And it's not unique to me, it's happening all over; many others are choosing to do this.

And so, where does that leave you now?
Let's find out.

PET WOULD BE THE WRONG WORD

You mentioned you're holding onto loneliness and pain; what's that from?
My major source is not associated with humans. I love humans and love them deeply, I work with them all the time - pet would be really a wrong word to use for humans, but I love them like a pet, and to understand them I must be them... And it's easier to be them when you start from the very beginning, from the fertilization, the exact thing that Michael Newton talked about,[85] going in and out as the embryo is developing, all those energies and bonding. It's atomic, it's chemical, it's hormonal, and an imprint - and you can mold that, you can literally create wonderful destinies for yourself, but when you come in... (Laughs) with that already in place! Yes, you may have had a bit of the design, but you weren't there experiencing it because you're off doing other things, so you're in for a shock, let's say - kind of like an earthquake; it tilts everything off kilter.

Because that life was geared for someone else.
Yes, and you've got to work with it, it's hard. I knew it would be hard.

Let's go back to the moment when you actually entered this body.
(Gasps and moans loudly.) I'm a complete stranger here, nobody recognizes me, I look in their eyes and they don't recognize me!

Is this the first time you've been in a human body?
I've been in many bodies.

---

[85] Referring to the experience many report in their LBL session of "going out and coming back" in while the fetus is gestating.

Explain why this is such an impact for you.
This is an intervention. (Sobs) Nobody really expected it; it was something planned very spontaneously. I intervened into this life.

So explain intervention.
It seems to revolve around my dad, my core family. Look at my list, everyone plays key roles. (Clients bring a list of friends and relatives in case they refer to them during their session, giving the therapist a reference point.)

And what's the connection between the two?
The human species has been closed, we have been reaching for the light, the great masters have come and gone, the messages have been received, we have been moved forward, and we are at a juncture. We must evolve, we must step to another level, a shift in our DNA, and light-workers among us are working passionately, furiously to get this to happen. Many people resist, we are not yet equipped; but those that are, are being led in dream states, many in trance states. There's an explosion of addictions; the reason why I'm involved (in my own) addictions is because I have to understand addiction, it's such an easy portal to go into, it's illusory, but it gives the semblance of the transformation which we all crave, which we stand on the brink of. That is the reason why we see so much, it is being revved up significantly, right now. Addictions are a trap.

A trap?
Folks are following their easy paths, which is why I have a body that's wired for addiction – to understand. I really love this planet so much, and it's so easy to get addicted to this planet, it's one of the most magnificent planets in all creation.

MOTHER EARTH IS SCREAMING FOR HELP

What makes it special?
It is intensely real; soulful. It has a humungous magnetic stream around it. This gives it energy and vibrancy, and yet it is so dense in its matter. The species that are on this planet, especially with brains large enough to connect to the light, have a joyous ride here, and manifest much. But we've gotten off track, because we've separated ourselves from our light and separated ourselves from our animal. We live in this void, yet we want to join and don't know how. And we're at war with ourselves, and at war with each other, and Mother Earth is screaming for help; she cannot tolerate it any longer. We all know this - so many of us are pouring in, which adds greater strain, but greater potential.

How does that add strain?
As population increases, the resources become more strained. We clamor to get each of our own, not knowing we have all that we need if we just share.

How many Earth lives have you lived?
Oh, thousands.

How old was this body when you first entered?
Four years old.

Tell me about the being that was here before you. About this agreement.

HIS SPIRIT GUIDE APPEARS

This being is in my soul group. (Gasps) Rhadime! Rhadime is one of my guides, a member in my soul group, a teacher; it's been a long time since Rhadime took physical form. But he took physical form for me, in this vessel (as a young boy), we co-created it, but he set some real challenges for me.

Let's talk to him right now.
Rhadime comes to me as a great eye. And then the eye transforms into different faces. He's a shape shifter, he's always changing, he's rather mirthful actually, that's where I get my playfulness.

Is he a peer? Or above you like a guide?
He's above me, he's a guide, but he's also my mentor, he's training me.

Let's call him forth to this session, if he will.
What would you like to ask?

Are you here with us?
(Voice audibly changes) We are here.

I'd like to know more about this body Thomas took over. That's pretty unusual...
It is not a common scenario. It's a scenario that Thomas desired. I needed to come forth, into his body to make the wiring, make those connections necessary for the path he was to take.

Why couldn't he do that himself, and why did you do that instead of him?
Thomas was incarnated in another body at the time this current body was born. He was going in the dream state and working in its development while living that life - it was important for him to come into this life to work with the beings that were incarnate at this time. If he remained in the life he was in, the chronology of events would have prevented him from being able to be present now.

Who and where was he in the life when you started this body?
He was here in the LA basin, he was in a woman's body - he died in his late teens. He was a she at that time. It was part of his transference difficulty, the melding of the male and the female, having not gone through that gestation period on the

spirit level other than in his dream state, was why he did not fully integrate. Also why there's always been confusion for him, which revolved around his sexuality. We knew this was going to be part of his reason before going to the path that he did, which brought him many detours and places of despair. But he needed to have a strong body, we worked together, I planted many seeds for him, which he has accessed at those important times. He has always known this, and it has brought him comfort, and brought him back into the path.

You asked why, it's just that this generation now, the beings that are incarnated now, the beings that will live now, the beings that will pass in the next 80 years or so, are going to be instrumental in the shifting of this planet; and the life work that Thomas needs to do could best be done in a vessel at this age, at this place and time, rather than the one he was in at the time of the transference.

What was he doing as a woman? What was he working on in that lifetime?
It was a carefree life, one of youth and abandon, comfortable means; a very joyful life.

What was his name?
Vicky.

What can we call Thomas' soul, so we don't confuse him?
Rhamanus.

So why did Rhamanus choose the Vicky lifetime?
It was a place of easy access for this life to go. When times get troubled, he's joyful and mirthful, not a care in the world; the quintessential easy life.

If the Thomas life is so important, why start another life ahead of it - when it's going to overlap? Why not just wait and start the Thomas life in the beginning?
Rhamanus has worked with the beings on that list,[86] as Vicky would never have made contact with them. It's important to note here that terms of grandiosity should not be built around this - because it's not – it was simply a matter of convenience. There are "walk-ins;" it's not common, often times great things come from them, but not necessarily things everybody knows about. It still has profound effects to the beings these intersections take place with.

If the Thomas life was so important to interact with these core beings in Thomas' life, parents, family and friends, why even start the Vicky life? Why not just wait?
It has to do with accessing those memories, because they mostly connect to the grounding spaces, the vortexes here on this planet. As Vicky, Rhamanus was surrounded by these vortexes, was in the energy fields. Many of the beings on the list were coming of age. So Rhamanus transferred that energy to Thomas.

---

[86] Referring to the list Thomas brought that he might reference during his LBL.

NOTE: "Grounding spaces" are reportedly parts of the planet that carry a higher vibration. Sedona, Arizona and Glastonbury, UK are two examples.

THE PARADIGM SHIFT

If Rhamanus started with the Thomas life, what would he have missed?
Opportunities. And healing. Opportunities and compassion. And having the joy of being part of the paradigm shift.

So what does Vicky bring to this soul of Rhamanus?
Vicky was a free spirit, she brings that to Thomas. I know this sounds complicated, but to simplify it, it comes down to if Vicky were alive today she'd be an older gal, she couldn't do the kind of work that Thomas could do with the key players in his soul group.

How does his soul group play a part?
We're all part of the same soul group - we have very different orientations however. They've all lived many incarnations in different roles. It is a gift for all three to be joined together during the present as great healing takes place in this life. It was worth the pain to make this happen, worth the transference; I am at peace for having done that, knowing it is okay.

So what is the focus of this group? Do they have a common work?
There is teaching on two levels; teachings of the heart and of love and acceptance. It's teaching diversity with a connection to the heart. With diversities in humans, there's often strife - diversity creates friction, creates imbalance, which creates physical maladies and degenerations. Most in this soul group tend to play healers. To one degree or another, disease often times manifests in the beings they choose, and as testament to their choice is the transformation that ensues as a result of it, whether it's teaching the opening of the heart or pathways to compassion.

They often choose difficult lives where lifestyles and cultures conflict, where there's a conflict of status and then they help to create bridges between the groups. It's an important time right now because bridges are being built everywhere, on this level and on other energetic levels. Think of this kind of healing work as a big 3 D canvas, with bridges of healing energy criss-crossing, with bridges coming above and below and through… criss-crossing to help people as they confront these cultural, societal differences.

A VISIT FROM A HIGHER SPIRIT GUIDE

So this group Rhamanus is in has around 8 or 9 souls? Does his group have an overseer or guide?
Valsoon.

Can Valsoon send us a message that would be valuable for Thomas today?
Stay connected consciously with your spirit guide Rhadime. Great work is to be done in the next seven years. Keep the faith and keep the strength, knowing all is well. We are proud of you.

Let me understand who Rhadime is. A guide?
He is a guide, transfers between this soul group, which is my primary soul group.

Can I have Rhadime speak as before? Would you address Thomas' questions now?
Yes, most of them.

Do you bring in other specialists or guides for Rhamanus?
We do, and did in his last transference to the ship. He was closer to the Valsoon presence at that time although they have actually never met.

What is the specialty that Valsoon has to give Rhamanus?
Valsoon is an overseer of evolution; he is one of the masters.

What is he giving to Rhamanus?
He teaches him fortitude, compassion. Because Thomas is more of a visitor to the human species than actually identified as such, it puts a very strange twist on things and oftentimes it becomes easy to be distracted from his primary purpose, which is to open up compassion and healing. This is Thomas's primary focus in this life, something he's known from the very beginning.

UNUSUAL DEFINITION OF THE HIV VIRUS

Tell us more about his mission in this life. You said compassion and healing?
As a carrier of a virus,[87] Thomas has a wonderful opportunity of walking through the transformative process, as an example. Using the restorative energies available on this plane to heal others by healing himself, his confusion in his connection to the previous life of Vicky and the DNA wiring of his life as a homosexual have created wonderful gateways to connections with other people - be they lifestyles, cultures, religions; it opens a natural compassionate portal. His struggle has been primarily about forgiveness; forgiving himself for lacking the complete integration when he came into this body, yet determined to work with the tools given to him. He needs to come to that place of forgiveness and that's why he called you. So that he could have this awakening on a conscious level and go forth from here, and the next seven years are primary in the work that is to be done.

---

[87] Thomas is HIV positive.

What does he need to do?
Thomas needs to align with those communities that are around him, that are also about the same thing. His new work in the Internet was so he could access those communities more fully.

What sort of communities?
Light-workers such as himself who are here to see the shift in the human species. It has been foretold for at least a generation; you've seen it in your pop culture, your songs, seen it in your prophecies, all humans on this planet can feel it. It's a vibratory state, it is a yearning. This planet has gone through several shifts; we are the brink of another. That is the community of which we speak.

Tell me more about the next seven years. What actions shall he take?
Keep the heart open, it will never lead you astray. That is Thomas's primary purpose, which he's become fully awakened to in the last year. He was scared, which is why he's come to see you today, Scott.

What's the main thing to come out of today's session?
He walks away with the assuredness he is on his path, fulfilling the destiny that he's contracted. He is aligning with the beings in his life and the ones coming into his life, that will be key instruments in helping him fulfill his contract. Never doubt and yes, he can heal AIDS in his body.

How is he to do that?
He is already doing it. He should continue what he's doing. It comes with the paradigm shift, and it's a DNA thing.

Can you talk about AIDS and why has it come to Earth?
AIDs is a metaphor that unifies the human species. It transmits; it's a being. It has its own realm of existence, one far greater than humanity, which comes through the act of making love on a species level. It's born of the oneness that is in everyone. The manifestation of degeneration and the attack to the immune system - the brave warriors who chose that path were those that showed the openings for people who were going to pass to the next plane very quickly. They brought the virus in great numbers, mainly through third world populations, through promiscuous populations; they came, they lived, and had brief, but intense lives; they served their mission and we thank them.

The HIV virus knits with the immune system, and the immune system is what keeps the physical species inherent. As soul beings, we are more than species, we know that in the shedding of these bodies we do not die; the fear of death is manifest in AIDS; and we can learn to not be afraid. The virus is a gift which helps us defeat our fear. The virus is encoded with DNA, DNA that is part of the shift of which we speak. It is not necessary to have this DNA shift through having HIV, but it is possible to have it with HIV; many can make the shift without it, many will, many are. A great many of those that carry the virus are light workers; they tend to be in the lifestyles of those that are shunned, those that are forgotten, and yet they show hope, love and compassion. They demonstrate we are one.

What percent of spirit energy is he using here and why?
Baseline is 45, sometimes it goes up to 85.

What does the other part of him do while this percentage is incarnated in Thomas?
He plays amongst his soul groups. He adds fortitude to its members. He is a playful sprite.

Why has he had so many challenges, constrictions and financial abundance issues?
Constrictions are self-perceived, they do not exist, they are projections; let the projections go. Abundance has always been here - be not tied to the abundance manufactured through the human means, it is yours for the taking. It comes in all ways, it has come in all ways, it is not linear. We do not have to adapt that stereotype, let it go.

Why does he feel financially constricted?
In this society, materialism is king. Power is through material gain. Identity that wraps itself around that stereotype is an illusion in the soul. There's great joy in dropping the projection.

Can you assist him to drop these projections right now?
This is planned, it is his contract, it is great work and we commend him, we honor him, it was a blessing to share this body for four years, we shared it together in the dream state when Vicky slept, much work was done together then.

You mean, when Thomas was 2 and you were in the body, Thomas would come and visit with you?
When Vicky was 15 and the Thomas body was one to four years old, in the dream states, yes.

So when Vicky was sleeping, Rhamanus would come and mingle with you?
That is correct.

Was there a purpose or a process?
There were lessons in learning to work with the adaptations in this body.

So you were schooling him how to work this body?
We were.

EXPERIENCING THE LIGHT

What is his deepest purpose in this life?
Love, heal, light. Always light. (Cries)

What are you experiencing?
A softness in my heart. Everything I do I feel in my heart. I know that I'm not alone but it hurts because it strings back to when I first got here, and those beings didn't recognize me, and I was alone.

You mean your family? They must have sensed a strange change in Thomas.
All beings sense that. There was a shift.

How did they relate to Rhadime?
Lots of frustration, the little infant crying, he couldn't stop.

Rhadime, why were you crying so much as an infant?
Colic was a big part of it. It was also the part of the vessel which had to be worked on for HIV. HIV responds mostly in the gut, so the development that was going on in the lymphatic at that time was profound, very elevated, very accelerated, for that little infant who was constantly in discomfort. Cried a lot, eventually had his tonsils taken out, just after the transference.

So this preparation was going on in 1960's when AIDS wasn't even known yet.
AIDS was here, but it was not yet known.

Did AIDS originate in Africa? Through monkeys?
It came through several portals; it is multi-species.

He asks "Why the addictions? The HIV?"
Part of the necessary wiring just to be able to relate to the energies going on in the species right now; you can never fully work something unless you honor it - until the tool becomes one with your hand, you never completely master the tool, never utilize it to its fullest.

A JOURNEY TO HIS HOME PLANET

Can you tell us about the home planet where Rhamanus lived his earlier lives?
It's a gaseous state; it's got bright whites and golds and oranges - infused with pinks. Think of a close-up of the Jupiter landscape, just swirling, you're not looking at it - you're in it.

Is it near to Earth?
It is in our Universe but it is so far, you need to inter-dimensionally transport. It's very far removed, in the farthest reaches of our ability to see.

Are we able to see the galaxy with our telescopes? Does it have a name?
It has a number. I'm seeing B-53 and Y-147[88]. Google it and see what comes up. (Laughs)

Tell us about life in that place. Is there a physical body?
It's not physically as dense as this, it's gaseous, and so it's easily permeable and malleable. It takes multiple forms - shape shifting, we resonate together...

A physical world, but a gaseous state. Is this world larger than Earth?
Much larger. Larger than Jupiter.

Does it revolve around a star? Do you know the name of the star?
Y-147.

Tell me about how people appear on this planet?
Thomas sees them in his sleep, they're ovoid. There's no sense of appendages, kind of like tails on the bottom. Eyes are very pronounced.

Kind of like eggs with tails?
Kind of, but much more elongated. There's pulsation, the way a jellyfish moves - like the gas is expanding and contracting. It emits gamma rays and other radiation, which is actually connected to the gas planet itself, think of the filaments in an anemone, each has its own eye, and there is one with the anemone at the base, one latched to the rock. These beings live this way.

Kind of flowing?
And connected to the planet.

Is this the most intelligent form of life on that planet?
(Laughs sarcastically.) They are very intelligent.

Why did you stop incarnating there and come to Earth?
The power of this planet is amazing, it offers transformation on the highest and the grossest levels; amazing deeds are done here. It is an honor to grow with this planet; the planet is an entity in itself. I am one of the workers, it is noble work, it is joyful, diligent and it spans the eons.

---

[88] The Andromeda Galaxy does have a star named NGC 147 (discovered by Louis D'Arrest). I can't decipher what B-53 might mean.

Back to Y-147. What's the name of the planet? Let's ask Rhadime. Does the planet have a personification?
Yes. All celestial beings have a life of their own. I'm getting jumbles of syllables. I see Morda-vere something, I get with this word the state of the gaseous planet itself, however it's unutterable in our vessel (as humans).

NOTE: As Thomas speaks via the voice of his spirit guide, it is markedly different than his own speaking voice, deeper, almost robotic. I had lunch with Thomas, interviewed him further, and found nothing in his background or present life which would connect him to this Yoda sounding, robot like persona. He had no idea what would come from his session, and certainly had no idea that I would be using it for the book. He had never met Scott, so there was no point in him being sensational for his benefit. Afterwards, he was as baffled by the concepts espoused during his session as Scott and I were.

THEIR MISSION ON EARTH

Let's just call it Morda. What do people do there?
Having transcended dense physicality, work and play are done. Our heavier state is the gaseous state, and the radiation states and those rays of energy go out into the celestial firmament, and the space ship which I'm talking about is but one of them. They're great explorers, they can go into realms that denser forms cannot because of their lighter form. And yet still retain physicality. Which is an experience different than being in the spirit realm, it's a wildly changing place, it's a very high dimension, and great work is done there. They are builders, they have sent Arks, many species have benefitted or been derived by their hands.

They seed planets? Do they work with DNA and the molecular structures of creatures?
Yes.

What's coming into your awareness?
Just the present moment of this space and time here now on Earth, and what's going on -- with disease and imbalance and the overpopulation and how prime we all are for a shift. The evolution curve is coming to its apex and a transformation will take place; it's been a long time in coming and it's happening now. It's an exciting time. We are all excited.

NOTE: This concept that Earth is in for a shift in consciousness has been put forth by numerous new age groups. However, interviewing Thomas I could find nothing in his background that would point him in this direction. He works as a landscape architect, is from San Francisco originally and has a successful business near Los Angeles.

THE STARSHIP FROM MORDA

Tell me more about this starship? Does it come and go?
It's always here but it pops in and out dimensionally, when certain things have to take place on a grosser level with the planet. It's always being monitored, guardianed, overseen.

Is it a physical structure? A metal sphere? Bullet shaped?
It's funny, I'm getting two things here; I'm getting a cylindrical ovoid shape, but I'm also getting like a gamma ray. And what comes to me is that Earth is being bombarded every second with gamma rays, which facilitates the presence of these beings, it's the highways upon which they travel. And they use that to pop in and out - when they pop in and out, there's is the semblance of physical structure, however I don't think it's physical as we know it, like it has some kind of metal alloy as we know it, I don't get that, I'm getting that it's more of a plasma.

How many others from Morda are here on Earth now?
Others as in other beings?

How many Mordans are here on Earth?
(Laughs.) "Mordans." Several hundred maybe. I see two ships, several hundred.

Are there any famous people that are from this same place?
Ohhhh, there are; we're not supposed to talk about that, not yet.

It just popped into my mind.
It's a good question and things pop into my mind when you say it. Some of them are driving filmmaking today, which wakens human consciousness, stimulates our fantasies and lifts us higher so we can then communicate. There are some social workers, who are making great strides, honestly though, the most power comes from the faceless, the going out and touching... wow... The touching. Now I get it.

NOTE: In my interview with Thomas afterward, I dug deeper into who he thought he was referring to during his session that might be working in film. He said he didn't have a clue. I threw out some names to him, wondering if perhaps he considered filmmakers who made stories about raising the consciousness of the planet might be part of his supposed group. I asked him to name the first person who came to mind. He said "Spielberg." I told him I knew the cinematographer Janusz Kaminski who is the cinematographer of many of Spielberg's films, and Mauro Fiore who shot "Avatar." He said "That rings a bell."

A SHIFT IN HUMAN DNA

Tell me about that.
Well the whole HIV thing, which of course comes through touching, sharing of blood life force, either through intercourse or the sharing of blood transmission - you're touching DNA together; there's one root. It's interesting, our species is so fearful of evolution and yet we aspire to it, and many times our evolution has been because of great travesty or what could be perceived as travesty. One species diminishes, another rises, one species dominates, eradicates the other; all have led to where we are now. We're on the brink of it again and it brings great fear. And yet it brings great transformation. We do not have to leave humanoid - humanoid does not have to be a forgotten tome in the dust, it can actually rise to the next level; that is what these workers are about.

What's the next level?
A shift in the DNA. When that shift takes place the spiritual portals we presently have in our auras and the ether, will become open and we'll be able to be in the physical and more connected to our spiritual. It's not an unknown thing here; there are plenty of people in history and present that have had this already.

Such as?
The mediums, the movement leaders who have certain gifts, they have a DNA structure that allow certain opportunities to come through their vessel the DNA shift. What we're talking about is on a grand scale, which will literally lift the species to its next level.

Let's talk to Rhadime about why there are two space ships.
One ship is in place when the other is not - think of an oscillation, think of a wave. They shift.

So one is always here.
From our human perception it would be a blink in, blink out, blink in, blink out. In other dimensions it could be great spans of time as we perceive it.

So there's usually a presence here?
Always a presence here.

Does it orbit the planet?
It does orbit.

Not detectable by human technology?
It has allowed itself in certain moments, these are usually anomalies perceived by the scientific instruments, and normally the oscillations are so fast that it's not recognized.

Was this a purposeful revelation? Or an accident?
It's not yet a revelation. When the species has evolved, when that DNA transformation has taken place, then the oscillations will be more readily perceived, and we'll have our ET visit for the first time.

You mentioned Rhamanus is affiliated with a second soul group. Let's check in on that second soul group. How many beings in the second group?
The two groups are delineated by their origination of home - the Mordans are one soul group and the rest on his list are in the other soul group and those beings would consider Earth their home.

(Reads the names of the rest on his list) So those are the Earth people?
These are spirit people, we all go to the same home, but they are about being human, and living the lives of humans, moving humanity forward, and moving their souls' evolution forward as humans; the Mordans are being human and evolving their souls as humans when they're human, but are doing it as ET's, does that make sense?

WHY THIS MESSAGE IS BEING DISCOVERED

Sure. Let me ask Rhadime if there is something else he'd like to show Rhamanus today, some place he needs to go, maybe a place of healing?
He actually has a message for you (Scott). He wants you to transcribe this. He wants you to meditate upon it. Because the work that you are doing is profound, it is a gateway for many, it helps connect, it's a fortitude, it's a restful place, it is a great honor what you're doing, and you've been given some new material that has not been written before; and you are worthy of having this, you are a good soul. You are a peace worker. It is an honor working with you and Thomas is blessed to be with you.

Thank you. Let me clarify, I shall transcribe some of this information, and do what with it now?
Meditate upon it, see what strikes chords in your heart, see if you're able to see parallels in others' experiences; we believe you will. The material that's been shared today goes beyond the "standard perception" of spirit being - the hierarchies described are of a divinity and there's a human link to divinity included in the passing and shedding of bodies. There are many opportunities for you in the next seven years to learn; try to be open.

Let me ask about your description of being a "walk-in" soul. It's not something we have been able to find in many other sessions.
As groundbreaking and noteworthy, commendable as this work is, there is more. Human beings are like filters, the planet is filled with filters, as we lighten, as we

shift, those filters will pass away, and the images will come more clearly with less distortion. You may consider that this was all farcical, somehow your (hypnotherapy) technique was flawed - you too must have fortitude, stand brave - in its right time, you'll present it. Be open. Look for connections.

Can you show Thomas something amazing or beautiful as a goodbye gift?
(He gasps loudly). I see my planet from far off and it's in a milky space and it's a bright white, creamy white, all of gas, in a very milky space and it's home and it makes me feel really good.

Which planet are you viewing?
It's my home planet. Earth is gorgeous too. But I can see my planet in the distance, pinned in a milky white field, and it's much brighter, it's not black, it's milky white, but it's a bright pin prick there.

So this is a place you've lived many lives.
Yes. Wow. No wonder I feel so outside sometimes. (Cries) Thank you for that.

How do you feel about what you've learned so far?
I feel that this has been a bold and a wild adventure and it connects those parts that have felt broken... and it provides validity for my life, who I am and what I'm doing. And I feel strengthened, and I feel awed.

Remember this loving world is always with you, take a deep breath, all your thoughts and memories will be retained and remembered to help you complete the remainder of your current lifetime... Etc. I'll count from one to ten and you can open your eyes..."
This session was controversial in many ways, especially for his claim that he was a "walk-in" – someone who showed up to enter into the physical form of a boy who was already 3 or 4 years old at the time. Dr. Newton has been asked about this; his research convinced him it doesn't happen.

I met Thomas in person after the session. Handsome, with an easy laugh and an engaging persona, I can attest he's not anything like the voice that came out of him during his session. When asked, he told me he had read a number of New Age tomes over the years, including Michael Newton's books. He had a number of ESP-like experiences as a younger man, and was familiar with the writings of the Urantia Book, which details beings from outer space being on Earth. For those skeptics out there, one could ask whether they influenced his session before he came in for it. I'll leave that up to you.

We discussed the possible meanings of his session – the suggestion there was some kind of tinkering with consciousness going on; he didn't know. He said he'd begun to meditate every day, and that his immune system had gotten better, much healthier than before his HIV exposure. He's positive and upbeat, and looking forward to whatever new revelations might come his way.

HIV ravaged the entertainment world in the 80's and 90's. To imagine they chose their lifetimes, knowing they'd go through suffering and pain is literally mind blowing. Upon their return home, according to this research, they'll be greeted like conquering heroes, who've helped humanity with their sacrifice.

People repeat these revelations as if it's something we need to pay attention to. Perhaps it's global warming, perhaps it's the health of humanity; perhaps it's the health of the planet. We're gaining this knowledge for some purpose, perhaps to further humanity, perhaps to save it from itself. But Thomas claimed that in the next seven years, an "ET" like event would occur on the planet, and he and his compatriots are here to pave the way spiritually for that coming event. An interesting prediction, to say the least. Would we be prepared for it, spiritually or mentally by then?

I believe things happen that can't be explained, but so many people seem intent on explaining them. Everyone has an answer for them. Either aliens or things from the spirit world.

- Harold Ramis

CHAPTER 19
MIND SCIENCE FOR A PROZAC NATION

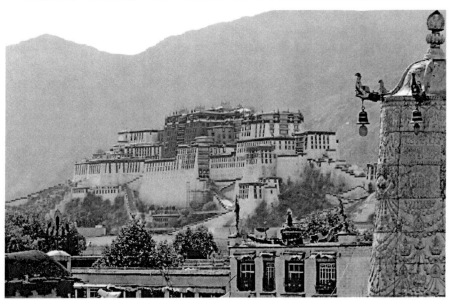

"I wouldn't consider myself a Buddhist or a card-carrying zealot at all. My first commitment is as a scientist to uncover the truth about all this... There are certain beliefs in traditional Buddhism that conflict with basic principles of scientific understanding... We can't make sense of those beliefs in any kind of scientific framework."

- Richard Davidson, University of Wisconsin.

As mentioned, when I was in Tibet, I traveled with Robert Thurman from Lhasa to Mt. Kailash where we did a trip around the sacred mountain. Robert had written a book about his first trip along with Tad Wise, which I picked up to read before I took my journey. "Circling the Sacred Mountain" had one passage in the book caught my attention, eerily reminiscent of my own volcano dream I had just prior to my friend Luana's death:[89]

"Suddenly, I felt surrounded by a buzzing, sizzling, roaring sounds, as if a gigantic rush of molten energy like a volcano was erupting within and all around. There was searing heat and yet I seemed to be in the perspective of the sacred mountain itself... A giant living crystal rock, aware of all of this within, yet completely free and still and cool. I felt an overwhelming surge of joyful giving toward all beings...Honey of life and happiness was flowing out of my crystal mountain's flaming void. Thunderbolt energy was crackling in all directions. A roaring, seething, hissing sound exploded all around."

As mentioned earlier, I had a similar "creation" vision where I felt like I was in a volcano, from a perspective of a platform of lava itself. I had the same experience of the roaring, buzzing, sizzling sounds. Did we both have a dream about the creation of the planet? When I read it in his book, I instinctively knew circling the mountain was something I'd do in this lifetime. Then oddly enough, the day came.

I was 15,000 feet above sea level, walking with my camera and backpack around this sacred mountain when I started hearing voices. My friend Paul Tracey had passed away only months earlier. A lifelong pal, he'd lost a battle with alcohol, and his mother sent me a mini-tub of ashes from his cremation. She'd sent a note saying Paul would have liked me to have them, and I kept them in a sacred place in our home in Santa Monica. Then, while planning this trip to India, and Tibet, as I was taking some of Luana's ashes with me, and I thought, "I might as well take Paul's too."

So while digging with a spoon in the plastic tub, I felt something. I found a steel ball about the size of a marble, and realized it was Paul's titanium hip – from the operation he'd had in high school that permanently damaged his hip, causing him to walk with a limp and cane for the rest of his life. Paul had been broken all the speed records in grade school, was a terrific athlete, and this operation had stopped him in his tracks. He spent the rest of his life dealing with one leg being shorter than the other, and later, a total hip replacement. It bothered him to no end, and may have been the source of his beginning battle with alcohol. As one friend put it, "The thing that Paul hated the most in his life, he willed to you."

I put the titanium ball in my bag and didn't think much of it until I was on the first leg of my trip around Kailash. *Damn, this is the hardest walk I've ever done in my life*, I thought. Walking in the Himalayas without knowing how to walk properly

---

[89] "Circling the Sacred Mountain" written by Thurman and Tad Wise. Bantam Books. Pg 338

can be extremely difficult. As it was, five of our group couldn't take the higher altitude and had to turn back. Suddenly I heard Paul's voice say "You think it's hard for you to walk? Imagine how hard it was for me all those years!" I stopped. I looked at the dirt cliffs surrounding me. Was I losing my mind?

"Paul, is that you?" "Yes," the answer came, as clear as bell. After a pause he said "You know, you were responsible for the happiest day of my life." I thought *what is he talking about?* And then, the image came to me; when we were 15 years old, we went on a trip to my uncle's home in Brecksville, Ohio. The head of the The Contractors Union in Ohio, A.J.P. Martini, owned a beautiful hunting lodge that overlooked the Cuyahoga river valley. A bigger than life character, he had this amazing ability to get people to gravitate to him, as well as wild animals. At sundown, he'd ring a huge ship's bell he'd gotten during his stint as a Navy "SeaBee" during World War II, (this is the Uncle who went to Burma and sent my dad a Tibetan thankga after the war) and all kinds of animals would come up the hill out of the valley to see what food he had to offer. He had a row of dog dishes lined up in his backyard, as the lightning bugs came out and lit up the night sky, wild animals would come out and dine in their dishes.

Pretty amazing sight for a kid from a suburb of Chicago; a half dozen deer, some raccoons and other animals, chomping on chewed up corn stalks, watching us as they peacefully ate together. One day Paul and I descended down the ravine in his backyard and followed the river. We got lost after a mile or so, and had no clue how to return. But we found a waterfall where large stones slabs sat atop an amazing pool of water. Paul and I dove from the slabs into the pool below for a number of hours. It was a magical day for two young boys to have, splashing and diving, not knowing if they'd ever make it home again.

Now here I was in Tibet, not having thought of that afternoon in some 30 odd years, and his voice inside my head reminding me of it. At some point I found a large stone "chorten," a Tibetan shrine stone pyramid made by pilgrims who'd brought a rock or two with them and planted Paul's hip in the center, within sight of Kailash's peak. So Paul's hip now holds up the center of a stupa which faces the sacred and magical Mt. Kailash, the mountain my son now calls "The wish mountain."

The second unusual event was after a long climb to the North Face of Kailash. The Sherpas helped set up camp, hot water and tea, and as the sun set about 4 p.m., there wasn't much to do after dinner. Robert began a fire ceremony, a six hour prayer session where his offerings to the deities of the mountains would ensure, as it had on three previous occasions, a safe journey around the mountain. I know it's effective, I've met more than one tourist who's attempted a trip around Kailash and been turned back due to bad weather. Even this would prove prophetic on this trip, as the Indian tour group behind us got caught in a sudden storm, and two of their tourists died from altitude sickness.

As I stood near him, watching him pray and helping toss wood onto the fire,

I closed my eyes and had an incredible vision – it was as if I stood next to a giant stream of energy, which moved, like a snake, or like the base of a tornado, and reached up into the heavens. My eyes were closed; I could see the twisting, pulsating energy stream and hear the rushing roar of it as well. Of course, you're up about 16,000 feet at that point, without oxygen, so one can always question what kind of things you see and hear.

But that night when I went back to my tent, I did my routine to make the tent a comfortable place to lay my head. A herd of yak walked nearby, their bells ringing in the most melodic tune I think I've ever heard. And as I was listening to their symphony, I heard another voice in my head, clear as a bell speaking to me in an English accent: "Richard. I think what you're doing is marvelous."

I thought, "Wow! At this altitude you really start to hallucinate!" I recognized the voice instantly, as the very distinctive voice of a famous actor that I only casually knew. It was the British stage and screen actor Michael Gough's distinctive voice. Michael had been a dear friend of Luana's for a number of years. She'd introduced me to "Mick" in New York, we went backstage to a Broadway show that he was doing, "Breaking the Code."

Luana was always a bit shy, and I insisted we go backstage after the show and say hello to her old friend she hadn't seen in years. There was a bit of a snafu, I don't think her name was given to him, and he was making his way home when we literally bumped into him in the darkness on stage. In the dim light, his jaw dropped, and he looked at Luana as if he was seeing the long lost love of his life.

He took us back to his dressing room and regaled us with stories; he and his wife Henrietta are two of the most wonderful people I've met. As of this writing, he's a spry 94, and Tim Burton uses him as much as he can - he's the voice of the Dodo in the new "Alice in Wonderland" film. He's starred in many films, including playing Batman's butler before Michael Caine took over the role.

I've met Mick a few times, and it was unmistakably his voice. But hearing someone's voice that clear outside a mountain in Tibet, I feared the worst. "Mick?? Are you dead?" I asked. "Oh no, darling," came his reply. "I'm here with Luana, and occasionally we take trips like this around the Universe, and I just stopped by to tell you that I think what you're doing, making this trip around Tibet, is marvelous."

It was as if he was in the tent with me. I had the sensation of seeing Luana hovering further back and away, and also the feeling she was having this adventure with him – and they both stopped on their "trip around the Universe" to see that I was in Tibet.

The first thing I did when I got back to the base of Kailash in Darchen, where there's an internet cafe, was to send Michael an email. "How... are you doing?" I asked. His wife Henrietta responded, "We're fine." It wasn't until a year later I reached him on the phone to tell him of the events of that night. I asked "Do you have any recollection of traveling in your sleep with Luana? Because I heard your voice while I was on Mt. Kailash in Tibet." He said "No, dear Richard, I have no recollection of that, but it sounds *absolutely marvelous*."

Once we made it around the mountain, we camped out on the shore of holy Lake Mansarovar. The water of the sacred lake is supposed to cleanse the soul, so a few of the intrepid campers took the opportunity to go for a splash. In my case I waited until it was about 4 a.m. when I waded into the ice cold water, dressed in only my skivvies, and sat. It was ice cold and I shivered as I splashed it over my head and around my body. It was there that I suddenly heard my father's voice say "That's enough!" I said "Ok, dad," and got out.

The next day I met an unusual pilgrim, "Swamiji." A young bearded Sadhu from India who speaks seven languages, he wears only a thin orange robe and no shoes. If you can imagine how hard it might be to walk over the stones along this high altitude lake, I was surprised at how he glided across stones I had a hard time navigating in my boots. I interviewed him about what he was doing on Lake Mansarovar; he said he walked there every year from his home in Delhi, India, and then walked back after spending six months living in a cave ("to check my email," he said with a smile). Sanjay Saxena, our tour guide, was with me as I interviewed him and we asked him to show us his cave. I've been told Swamiji has become a major holy man in both India and Tibet, and people line up for hours to meet him.

Sanjay and I went up and sat in his tiny, mountain retreat. Swamiji has a spectacular view of this sacred Crystal Lake Mansarovar - once outside the wind, it was calm. He pulled out a book from his robe - a coffee table sized picture book filled with pictures he'd taken of the upper regions of Mt. Kailash. A German cameraman had left him film and cameras, and while he took his trips atop Mt. Kailash (clad only in his robe) he'd taken these amazing photographs of a part of Earth people rarely get to see. I asked him if the German cameraman had given him any royalties from his work on the book. He smiled and said, "And what would I do with them? Look around. Do I have room for any more stuff?" It was true; he had only enough room for a few utensils and a teapot. I made him an offer; "Look, I live in a cave in Santa Monica. We call it an apartment. Let's trade caves. You come and live in my cave, and I'll live in yours, let's see who lasts longer;" nothing quite like making a holy man belly laugh.

All of this started with the coin flip. I was trying to decide if I should live in Rome or come back to the states. I pulled out a 100 lire coin; heads I would stay in my beloved Roma, tails, I'd seek my fortune in Los Angeles. I flipped it, allowing the fates to dictate what my life would be. It came up heads. I thought "Oh shit, two out of three." That made me realize I probably should go to L.A. Then 25 years later, when my daughter Olivia was born, I dreamt about the coin flip. I could see clearly that every move in my life had been plotted out like an elaborate chess game, from the coin flip to her birth. And If I hadn't flipped that coin in a train station in Rome, I wouldn't have gone to USC film school, met Luana, wound up making films, traveling to India to make a Bollywood film, conveniently close to Nepal where I got to take this trip of a lifetime filming Robert Thurman's trip around Mt. Kailash - nor would my son have been able to find me on that sacred mountain. But what's the mechanism behind this elaborate chess game of life?

TRAINING THE BRAIN THROUGH MEDITATION

It's all in the mind.

They say atoms have a tendency to find other atoms they're familiar with. Quantum Physics tells us if one set of atoms is familiar with another set of atoms, when you separate the two, they have a tendency to find each other again. Further, if you stimulate the first set of atoms in one place, the atoms that were separated tend to react to the same stimulus, the way twins react when one is in danger or in fear. In some of the sessions I filmed, under hypnosis, people would say that we are all interconnected, like a symmetrical array of sparkling lights, and that the energy of the Universe flows through all of us. Is it possible when someone finds themselves in a situation that seems coincidental; it's not coincidental at all?

I was invited to attend a lecture of Richard Davidson, who was going to discuss his latest findings on meditation at UCLA. Time Magazine called Davidson one of the 100 most influential thinkers of our time. [90] His work began at the University of Wisconsin in Madison where he began to study the effect of meditation on the mind using rigorous blind testing models and subjects who had a history of meditation.

In order to get into his study, a person had to prove they'd had at least 10,000 hours of meditation, basically a year and a half sitting in a lotus position. They agreed to a battery of lab tests which would prove or disprove the benefits of meditation on the human mind. The results were revolutionary.

In his lecture at UCLA, Davidson spoke to a room full of psychiatrists and psychologists, looking for alternate methods for treating depression in their Prozac nation. Davidson's work shows meditation can actually change the structure of the brain to make a person happy. Even one session can affect the physical shape of the amygdala, the part of the brain which monitors depression. When Time magazine did their article on his work, they showed a Tibetan monk whose response was off the charts; the caption was "The Happiest Man on Earth."

But Davidson's work shows anyone can benefit from meditation. Depression can be cured, and patients can get off medication by learning the proper techniques. Parents who enroll children in a yoga class have a statistically better chance at making them happy, rather than through medication.

There are numerous Tibetan meditations, some are very precise as to what steps or thoughts should be employed, and I asked Dr. Davidson what he'd used for his survey. He told me "Tonglen."

---

[90] The Time 100 - People Who Shape Our World. April 30th, 2006

Tonglen is a meditation Tibetan monks use to cure people or the planet of its ills. A Tibetan doctor or Lama might use it to heal a patient. Specifically the meditator pictures the patient sitting across from them, seeing them from head to toe; hair, eye color, their smile, every detail possible.

Then the meditator pictures the affliction - heart, mind, perhaps an inflammation or even cancer – and then breathes in, pulling the illness with their breath, into themselves. Once they've pulled it inside, they bathe it in a healing light - some call it "the healing light of the universe" But a bright light that pulverizes the illness. The light dissolves the illness and turns it into a bath of white, healing, healthy energy - and with their out breath, they breathe that healing, positive light back into their patient.

Dr. Davidson's asked his subjects to do a "universal tonglen," as he didn't want to skew the results by having each meditator consider a particular individual, but the planet as a whole.

One interesting result is that even if the patient isn't cured, the meditator feels physically better. Apparently the study shows that the act of compassion actually changes your own brain structure, this compassionate meditation brings about profound changes in the amygdala of patients. One session of Tonglen, according to Davidson's research, can profoundly affect your life.

Here's an excerpt from the study:

Meditative instruction

"During the training session, the subject will think about someone he cares about and let his mind be invaded by a feeling of altruistic love or of compassion toward these persons. After some training the subject will generate such feeling toward all beings and without thinking specifically about someone. While in the scanner, the subject will try to generate this state of loving kindness and compassion."[91]
And the results, as published:

Abstract

Recent brain imaging studies using functional magnetic resonance imaging (fMRI) have implicated insula and anterior cingulate cortices in the empathic response to another's pain. However, virtually nothing is known about the impact of the voluntary generation of compassion on this network. To investigate these questions we assessed brain activity using fMRI while novice and expert meditation practitioners generated a loving-kindness-compassion meditation state... The comparison... showed increased activation in amygdala, right temporo-parietal junction (TPJ), and right posterior superior temporal sulcus (pSTS) in response... Together these data indicate the mental

[91] Lutz A, Brefczynski-Lewis J, Johnstone T, Davidson RJ (2008) Regulation of the Neural Circuitry of Emotion by Compassion Meditation: Effects of Meditative Expertise. PLoS ONE 3(3): e1897. doi:10.1371/journal.pone.0001897

expertise to cultivate positive emotion alters the activation of circuitries previously linked to empathy and theory of mind in response to emotional stimuli.[92]

Dr. Davidson reported the amygdala, associated with depression, actually changes shape during the meditation. Combining meditative music and thought, they were able to prove that this form of meditation can help cure depression. In a nutshell, by using your mind, you can cure depression.

How does this relate to the Afterlife?

People under hypnosis report visiting healing centers where they use energy to cure all manner of ills that they might have experienced during life. In the afterlife, people use energy to heal people. In my own session, I claimed I visited a classroom that was teaching people in the spirit world, how to help healers on Earth to manipulate energy so that it helps their work to be more effective. That is, helping a doctor, or healer, or surgeon while they're at work, so the results are positive. And according to Davidson's research, training the mind to tap into this healing energy of the Universe is also a way to benefit humans - it actually affects the person doing the meditation to become healthier, more relaxed, and in the case of depressives, to change their outlook of the planet altogether.

Toss away your prescription for Prozac and Zoloft and pick up a book on how to meditate. At least you can save yourself a bundle![93] But how does an energy pattern in the mind relate to consciousness?

In terms of Tibetan treatises on the ability of the mind to control consciousness, one of the most famous is the "Six Yogas of Naropa." This esoteric tradition in the Tibetan lexicon - it comes from the yogas that a pandit named Naropa had perfected. I won't go into the details of Naropa's story; it's fascinating, bizarre, but at some point, Naropa began teaching mental exercises to his pupils, and those yogas were passed along from teacher to student by word of mouth for centuries. Actually it wasn't until just a few years ago, when Buddhist leaders allowed for the publication of the yogas, that anyone could have seen them in English.

These yogas are mental exercises for the brain that deal with transferring energy into various places in and outside of the body. Most people have heard of various energy centers in the body – chi, or the chakras, for example – these yogas describe focused meditations that include transference of this energy into inanimate objects, even recently deceased animals. An example cited was a Buddhist masters taking a dead bird, and getting it to fly again.[94] Also included is the practice of *tummo* -

---

[92] Lutz A, Brefczynski-Lewis J, Johnstone T, Davidson RJ (2008) Regulation of the Neural Circuitry of Emotion by Compassion Meditation: Effects of Meditative Expertise. PLoS ONE 3(3): e1897. doi:10.1371/journal.pone.0001897

[93] Obviously Prozac and other psychotropic drugs help people; else they wouldn't be so popular. But could a little meditation hurt?

[94] "Tsongkhapa's Six Yogas of Naropa" translated by Glenn Mullin. This is a commentary on the various yogas.

commonly practiced by Tibetan monks as part of their graduation ceremony.[95] Monks are sent out in their light robes into a snowy bank, where wet towels are brought out and put around their shoulders. While they're sitting in the snow, they create the *tummo* inner fire - and the resultant "mental flame" actually brings the temperature of the monk to a much higher level. I've seen footage of monks doing the exercise, where steam comes off the wet towels as they're placed over the monks' shoulders. It's literally mind over matter; in this case, the body's structure.

I have a friend who is an acupuncturist in New York. She spent many years training as a massage therapist as well, and told me that when she was involved in a session, she'd frequently pick up visuals of the person's life she was working on. She could accurately recount to them episodes in their life, almost as if the stress from those incidents remained, energy-wise, in the muscles she was unwinding.

Carlos Castaneda adopted R. Buckminster Fuller's concept of architectural integrity called "Tensegrity" to describe the philosophy he claimed to have learned from Yaqui Indian Don Juan who described the universe as being devised of energy, and organized by a force of intelligence. There are practitioners who use intent and their hands to adjust and reform the energy of patients who come for this unusual form of therapy to this day. These same energy portals are claimed to be identifiable in yoga, in Asian medicine, Tibetan medicine in particular.

The chakras, life force or chi, the energy flow of a human body is quantifiable, and from what we've seen in this research, may contain memory packets from previous lifetimes. So it would make sense that if a person was out of alignment, energy wise; their physical form would suffer as well. Yoga, meditation and other mental exercises can help realign a body's energy, both mentally and physically. Meditation is proven to affect the mental process, a verifiable cure for depression and other mental illnesses.

So it is possible with specific training, for the mind to physically alter the energy of the body. This is also apparently true with healing practices, unconscious or otherwise.

Some years ago, there was a story on National Public Radio about research[96] done about psychosomatic illnesses, and people who could create unusual illnesses only with their multiple personality minds. In one case, when a person slipped into another personality, that persona had hives, and the patient would break out with them. In another case a little African American girl had stigmata, and although not being Catholic or from a religious family, would bleed through her palms and feet. Oddly enough, it's fairly accepted that Jesus would have had to have been nailed in his wrists in order to keep him on the cross, but the psychiatrists involved with the case were convinced the little girl had imagined it herself, and brought the stigmata to herself based on something she must have seen on television. And finally, one

---

[95] See "Mind Science" by the Dalai Lama and others, listed at the end.
[96] http://en.wikipedia.org/wiki/Tummo

of the people examined who had multiple personalities, one of the people he imagined himself as had a lazy eye, or a wall eye. Imagine for a moment the tricks the mind would have to do to convince the muscle in the eye to wander, and only when this alternate persona appeared in the mind. Here's an excerpt from a Bill Moyer's interview of Candace Pert about Multiple Personality Disorder:

Candace Pert, PHD: Emotions are in two realms.[97] They can be in the physical realm, where we're talking about molecules whose molecular weight I can tell you, and whose sequences I can write as formulas. And there's another realm we experience that's not under the purview of science. There are aspects of mind that have qualities that seem to be outside of matter. People with multiple personalities, for example, sometimes have extremely clear physical symptoms that vary with each personality. One personality can be allergic to cats while another is not. One personality can be diabetic and another not.

Bill Moyers: "But the multiple personality exists in the same body. The physical matter has not changed from personality to personality."

Candace Pert: "But it does. You can measure it. You can show one personality is making as much insulin as it needs, the next one, who shows up hour later, can't make insulin."

In "The Holographic Universe," Michael Talbot quotes a number of sources of people who discuss psychosomatic illnesses that are manifested in multiple personalities. He writes of people who are allergic to a food or substance that one of their personalities is not allergic to.[98] He goes into details about patients who've cured themselves from a variety of diseases by using meditation fully on their health system.

From Joseph Campbell: "It is part of the Cartesian mode to think of consciousness as being something peculiar to the head, that the head is the organ originating consciousness here in the body. The whole living world is informed by consciousness. I have a feeling that consciousness and energy are the same thing…. Where you really see life energy, there's consciousness… The whole process is consciousness. Trying to interpret it in simply mechanistic terms won't work."[99] It's the same structure at play that we learn about the Na'vi in the film "Avatar;" all the biodiversity in the cosmos is energetically connected, interdependent, working together to give us life. Consciousness may reside in some place outside of our bodies in the energy ether of the Universe, and we use it, as Gary Schwartz describes it in the Foreword, the way a radio uses an antenna.

All the years we've been on the planet, no one has been able to quantify or define what consciousness is. They can't point to when it appears, or if and when

---

[97] Excerpt from Healing and the Mind © 1993 by Public Affairs
[98] Pg 98 "The Holographic Universe." Dr. Howland, a Yale psychiatrist recounted a patient who came in with a swollen eye from a bee sting, but under hypnosis, the swelling disappeared, only to recur when the other personality returned.
[99] Joseph Campbell The Power of Myth © 1988, Doubleday

it goes. They can point to people who don't seem to have it; people in a coma perhaps, or severely injured, or having a physical affliction - but even then, it can't be proven they don't have consciousness. And there's been quite a bit of speculation, especially in the world of quantum physics, that energy of the body might actually be part of consciousness.

"What is mind?" "What is matter?" and how does mind have an effect, if it does, over matter? If a person can focus their mind to make depression disappear, to make physiological changes in the body, then what, or who is controlling the mind? Buddhism teaches there is no finite self; what we perceive as "I" is actually a relative self, one ever changing. That if you slice through all the levels of gross matter, sensation, memory, etc, that at the end of that examination one winds up with nothing, or emptiness. Or the space between atoms, to put it in another fashion.

But is this actually the case?

If it's true energy can't be destroyed and also true that no matter where one takes an atom from one energy group into the universe, the ones left behind will react whenever the other is stimulated. As mentioned, atoms have a tendency to seek each other out again, no matter where the other atoms have gone. The same principals seem to be at work in our spiritual selves.

What if we can tap into the ability monks or people with multiple personality disorder have demonstrated? Could the mind help the body eliminate disease or psychological blocks? Is it possible a hypnotherapy session could cure a phobia or fear or illness that's been traveling with us for many lifetimes? Is it possible if I'd discovered this information years earlier I might have been able to save Luana's life? Or did she choose to go through the incredibly difficult process in order to learn and benefit from those difficult spiritual lessons?

It was time for me to try a return visit to the life between lives. A second session would confirm the research I'd been doing, and would help confirm other details. Had I really seen her in the life between lives, and with the help of a different hypnotherapist, on the other side of the country, would I be able to find her yet again?

*"You would know the hidden realm where all souls dwell.
The journey's way lies through death's misty fell.
Within this timeless passage, a guiding light does dance.
Lost from conscious memory but visible in trance."*

- Michael Newton

CHAPTER 20
THE EYES OF JESUS

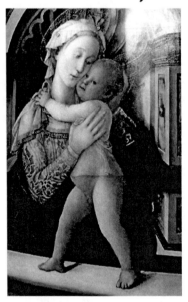

He changed sunset into sunrise.
- Clement of Alexandria

A friend told me of some recent trauma in her life. She'd lost her mom, lost her job, and felt at her wit's end about having to sell her home and move back to her native Pennsylvania. A vivacious blonde in her early 60's, "Molly" has seen it all during her sojourn in Hollywood. As well as being an accomplished actress, she's been a personal assistant to some of the most famous people in Hollywood. I sat with her and described the kind of soul work I'd been researching, how it showed that even trauma could be to our benefit, and that our departed loved ones aren't really gone. She said "I want to do a between life session, now!" I called Scott de Tamble to see his availability and we recorded the following session at Molly's home about a month later.

Scott: (after 30 minutes of deepening) Let's go back to the stairway now... going younger and younger... five, then four, down, down, younger now, smaller and smaller, three, two... one... 6 months, back to the womb. How does that feel?
Molly: It just feels dark.

Tune into her heartbeat.
I feel like I can't breathe.

Let's go back a little further, a little younger, where you feel comfortable.
(Sighs) Better.

I want you to tune into your mom.
She's with my brother Billy. She loves him.
  NOTE: Prior to the session I learned a couple of things from Molly before Scott arrived; one was that she had a brother Billy who died young, and also that she was born not breathing. After her father accidentally dropped her, she gasped and came to life.

Can you move your awareness outside your mom?
(Nods) Uh-huh. My dad's in the Air Force so he's away. I feel this worry from my Mom. I just feel the worry.

Do you attempt to comfort her? Or are you just observing?
I feel I'm staying back.

At what month did you join the fetus?
Seven comes to mind.

What about the brain and body? Your first impression.
I feel small and weak. I just don't feel much. I don't feel connected.

Do you feel like you have a problem with making a strong connection?
It's like (it's) lost, I can't find it. The connection.

Does it feel like the soul is holding back? Or the body?
The body.

Let's tune into this little body and see why it's holding back.
Numb, I just feel numb. My hands are tingling.

If the body could talk, have it tell us why it doesn't connect.
All I sense and feel is the weakness. I feel… I just hope she wants me.

Do you feel she does or doesn't want you?
She's scared, having two kids. (Billy is 16 months older) My dad's in the Air Force; he's in Dover. She's alone.

Does that affect you in some way?
I think I feel affected. I can't help her. I want to help her, but I can't because I'm little.

How are her emotions affecting you?
They're making me afraid.

There's fear and worry that makes your body feel weak?
Yeah.

Now that you understand that, things will be different in the future. Let's move away from this time in the womb, float up and away… As I count from five down to one… Step into a tunnel that leads to your own past… Be there now. Is it daytime or night?
Night.

Inside or outside?
Inside. Lying down. I'm alone. I'm comfortable.

What's the surface like?
It's soft. Lying on my back.

Male or female?
Female. A small person. Young.

What's the age?
8. I'm an 8 year old girl.

Where are you?
It feels like people are dancing. Grownups, in simple clothes. Everyone's holding hands.

What are you wearing?
Cotton. Like a dress. Like brown paper color. Barefoot. My hair is long, flowing, brown. I'm outside now, I'm dancing. I'm looking for a hand to grab. There's music.

How do you feel?
Happy.

Tell me about her face, her complexion?
It's fair. She's cute. She has light colored eyes; blue.

Look through those eyes and connect with this girl. What's your name?
I don't know.

We'll come back to that. Is it night or day?
It's day now.

Are you still 8?
(Shakes head, no.) I don't know. It's confusing.

Just be there enjoying the dancing. Feels good?
(Nods) Uh-huh.

While you're dancing, I want you to go back in time in your mind, the little girl's mind and picture the place where she lives. Let that come into your mind.
I'm starting to feel really anxious, like panicked.

Tell me more about that.
I just want to get away.

Ok, as I count down from three, go back in time and see where her home is. Where do you sleep?
It's simple. Not much of a place to lie down. It's a tent.

What's inside the tent?
Just blankets.
    NOTE: She later described the tent as small, but big enough for her to stand in.

As I count to three go to when you're enjoying a meal. What are you having?
Bread… and fish. Just water to drink.

Is there a drinking vessel?
Bowls.

What part of the world are you in; a name, a place, a continent?
Jerusalem.

215

What is the year that you're experiencing?
I see 18.

Is there something before or after the 18? Is that before or after Christ, is that A.D. or B.C.?
I just see 18.

I'm going to lift your hand, let it be loose, your name as this little girl is going to come to you. Three, two, one...
June.

As I count to three, I want you to go to a very proud moment in your life as June. One, two, three... be there now.
I'm outside. I'm aware of other people and I'm in front of them.

How old are you?
Older. 20. I'm standing alone.

Why is this a proud moment for you? As they look at you, what's in their eyes?
Joy.

What are you wearing?
White.

Like a white dress, tunic or something?
(Nods) Uh-uh.

Does it feel like a special occasion?
Everyone's happy.

How do you feel?
Scared. I think I'm getting married...

Is this the ceremony?
There's no man, I don't see any man... I just see these people.

What happens next?
Maybe it's a play. Maybe it's acting. Feels like it. But there are no words. Like a performance.
    NOTE: Later, she observed that it might have been a "baptism."

Where are you?
I'm still in Jerusalem.

You said the year is 18 something... is this the time when Jesus is alive, or before or after that?
Jesus is alive.

Have you ever met Jesus or seen him?
I think so.

As I drop your arm I want you to go to that moment when you behold Jesus; one two three. Be there now. Where are you?
In a large crowd. Outside.

How old are you?
My 20's.

What's going on? Is a crowd milling about?
They're listening. Someone's preaching.

How far away are you from the person talking?
About ten feet.

What's that person's name?
John comes to mind.

What's John talking about?
He wants... he keeps saying "Listen." I only hear "Listen."

What does he look like?
Not so tall; medium. He's thin. Has long hair, past his shoulders. It's flowing, lot of flowing hair. It's wavy. Color is dark brown. He's Bearded. Same color as his hair. Beard not so long; he's handsome.

How's the crowd responding to him?
Quietly. Patiently. Seriously.

Like he's saying something important...
Yes.

What's his full name?
I.. it makes me want to laugh, but I keep hearing "John the Baptist."

Is this a common occurrence in this part of the world, people out talking?
Yes, it's common.

Is this more special or rare, this guy? A celebrity or something?
He's important.

People are taking this to heart?
Yes.

How large is the crowd?
Hundreds.

What does John stand on?
He's standing on something. I don't know what it is. It's like a village where the tents are.

How do you feel?
I don't feel like I live there. I'm traveling, I'm just there.

Do your people travel a lot?
I feel like we're travelers.

Where is this?
It still feels like Jerusalem.

Tell me about your people, you way of life.
Always moving; we're gypsies.

How do they make their living?
Jewelry.

Do you see any other people talk? Have you ever seen Jesus talk or preach?
Maybe.
    NOTE: She later told me that June felt resistant to speaking about the following topic.

If you've ever seen Jesus in the flesh, I want you to go to that scene, as I count from three to one. Be there now. If you've ever seen Jesus, the Christ in the flesh in this lifetime as this gypsy traveling girl, I want you to be there. And if not you can just go to some pleasant scene in her life. So what's coming into your mind?
(Starts to speak – doesn't.) I feel mesmerized.

Tell me more.
I feel I can't... I can't believe what I'm seeing.

Let go of that, and flow into what you're seeing and tell me about this. What are you seeing? Inside or outside?
I'm outside.

Alone or with others?
There are others.

Just describe what you're seeing.
I do see the face of Jesus.

What's going on in this scene?
He's speaking. I'm just mesmerized.

What is it about him that mesmerizes you so?
His purity. His honesty. His heart.

So you're able to perceive these qualities?
His truth.

Tell me about his face.
Beautiful. I almost can't breathe.
    Allow his purity to calm you, his truth to relax you. It's okay. Imagine I'm a blind person, I want you to describe his face for me. What about the shape?
    Narrow. Clean. Soft. Intense.

What about his color?
Tan.

Is it olive skin? Ruddy? Dark? Fair skin?
(Shakes head.) Tan. Just tan.

His face is narrow and tan. Tell me about his hair.
Simple. Long and simple.

Is it thick or thin?
Thin. It's light brown. Shoulder length. Wavy.

What about his eyes?
They're brown, a golden brown.
    NOTE: Later she said that "clean" meant he didn't have a beard, his face was tan, as opposed to olive colored. Biblical scholars have debated that the father of Jesus may have been a soldier or someone named Pandeira, as he was referred to as "ben Pandeira" or son of Pandeira, whoever that may have been. But it might account for a fairer, or more "northern" complexion. She later told me she was standing "only a few feet" from him as he spoke.

I want you to etch this in your mind for all time, I want you to be able to go back to this scene in your mind. You'll remember this forever.
(Cries)

What is that you're feeling?
Such love.

Where do you feel that? In your body?
Everywhere (Cries).

Feel that, breathe it in. What else do you feel?
Humbled.

Tell me about the clothing of Jesus.
Brown. Different layers and pieces of clothing. Much of the same color.

Is he wearing a robe or tunic?
Robe.

Anything on his head? Feet?
Bare head, I just see his bare feet.

While Jesus is talking and you're feeling these feelings, what is he speaking of?
Love.

What is he saying about love?
That you *must* love. I just feel his kindness. It feels like the way it should be.

The kindness feeling?
Yes.

His words and presence really have an effect on you, don't they?
Yes.

Are you sensing that he's different from other speakers?
He's different.

How do the other people with you feel? Mesmerized?
Yes.

Just be there in his presence, drinking in his beauty and purity, take it into you. Let it transform you.
(Sighs)

Let's move forward to the end of the talk, what happens? Where does he go?
He just walks away. I go back to the tent.

Do you talk to anyone about this?
No. I'm just wondering where he will be next, so I can see him again.

Let's go to the very last day June is alive, not yet have crossed over. Are you inside or outside?
Inside. Lying down. I'm 80 years old.

Go back to that day when you saw Jesus preach.
(Cries) He was my friend.

What do you mean by that?
I knew him. He was a friend to my people. He showed us how to live. How to love. To be good. To be kind. To be honest.

What happened to him?
He died.

Were you there? Or did you just hear about it later?
I couldn't see, I couldn't watch.

What happens to him?
He was killed. They beat him and tortured him. (Cries)

Did you know this was happening?
I couldn't take it.

You were present when this was happening?
I was near. It was my people that he watched and took care of.

I don't understand, could you be more clear?
Our friends, our family. He helped us.

By teaching you how to live?
To love and be kind.

And now he's being tortured and killed?
He's dead.

How do you know he's dead if you weren't watching?
It's what they say.

When you say he "helped your people," who are your people?
(Shakes head.)

A traveling people? You lived in tents?
Yes. Gypsies.

So he was a friend to your people?
Yes. He taught us how to live, how to love.

From when you saw him preach, how long of an interval goes by until he dies?
Years. Five comes to mind.

So let's go to your last day. What's going on with you? You're not feeling too well?
Tired.

What do you think about this life?
It was hard.

What was hard about it?
Everything.

Without pain or discomfort, it's time to move to the moment after death, so when I count to three, you'll have passed over. One, two three… you've been through this many times before, I want you to rise from your body, free… Where are you in relation to your body now?
I'm in the dark. I feel tingly. I feel pressure in my chest. Like someone's sitting on it. It hurts.

Where is that coming from?
My heart.

Is this physical or emotional pain?
It's heavy. I don't think she's died yet.

She's feeling that heavy pressure in her chest?
(Nods)

I'm going to lift your hand, as I drop it, let her pass over, let it all go - let her die, and you can pop right out of the body feeling really good, free, pleasant. One, two, three. How's that feel? Better?
Grateful to be out of there.

What did you learn from that lifetime?
To be good.

Anyone you want to say goodbye to?
Just goodbye. Bye bye.

All right… your soul can feel the joy of being released from that life because you've been this way before. Anything you need to do before leaving?
Just to say "Thank you."

How do you feel?
Like my head's about to bust wide open.

Okay, moving up and away now, your vibration getting higher and higher... etc. How are you feeling?
I feel as if my head is opening up. I sense twinkling. Twinkle lights like…

Move towards those lights.
(Sighs) It's like when my mom died in my arms, and I held her, it feels like that light. It's like a fog light, but brighter.

How does that make you feel?
It makes me feel like I felt when my mother died and I let her go. (Cries)

How would you describe that?
I wanted to go with her.

This is a time when we can make a visit.
I'm just remembering my mother.

What about the twinkling lights?
There's less twinkle and more light.

Connect with this light now, move right into that light, connect with it, is this a person, or is this just a force. What is this?
Just at peace. Peaceful. It's gotten a little darker.

How are you feeling now?
Safe.

What are you experiencing?
I just feel I'm with my mom.

Is she embracing you?
It's so intense. It's almost too much. She's with my brother and my father, I feel like they're here. Pretty scary.

I want you to embrace them.
I feel like I'm getting a migraine.

Tell your mother you get the message.
"I get it mom."

Let's ask her to remove the headache.
"Mom I get it, I can't do anything about my hair."

Give her a hug and ask her to remove your headache.
"I love you mom." (Sighs)

What about your father?
He's with me all the time.

You can communicate with him now if you want. What about your brother? You need to communicate with him?
Billy, Billy, Billy…

I want to ask Billy if he has a message for you… speak that message aloud so it gets on your recording.
He said he's sorry. (Cries)

What is he sorry about?
He wasn't clear what he wanted for my Mom. For not being clear.

Anything else he needs to tell you?
He always told me, "Not to feel guilty and to enjoy my life."

Is he reminding you of that now?
Yes.

What about your father?
He told me that he loved me and he was never able to do that until I was forty years old when I finally made him tell me. Because I needed to hear the words.

Let's tune into your mom. Let see if she has a message today.
All I hear is "How was your son's graduation?" "It was great, mom. It was good."

Any other messages?
I just miss 'em.

You can be with them again, right now, embrace them in that family hug. Your heart can say all those things that you feel.
"Keep your eyes on my son." I'm telling them.

What do they say?
They know.

Ask your mom to take us to a place where you need to go.
I just feel so heavy from these feelings.

Let's ask her to take you to a place of healing, a special place. What's coming into your mind?
I'm breathing easier.

Let's go to a place of healing. Be there now.
I feel like I'm in a box.

Floating?
I'm lying down. Feels like an oxygen tent.

Good, take a deep breath. You need more time in this box?
Maybe a little.

Ask in your mind to be led to your guide, or ask your mother to guide you. Just open your mind and be there. Is it a male or female energy?
I feel a male.

What's the first thing that comes through from this person?
"Be safe."

What are you aware of?
I just feel a presence and an energy. It's electric. I feel like the electricity's going through me, not tingling, just like an energy. It just took a lot of the pain out of my legs. It feels like it's filling me up. -- He just told me to breathe.

What should we call this energy?
I always call it Hal, not sure if it's the right name, but Hal works for me.

So what is Hal communicating to you about the past life we looked at? As June?
It's like he knew. Maybe he was there too. It feels like he knew June.

Was he incarnate during that time, alive? Or was he June's guide then as well?
He's laughing. He was there. I don't hear an answer, but I sense that he was there.

Let's make this easier, I'm going to speak to Hal directly, is that okay?
He's still laughing.

Hal, what was the reason to show her this lifetime today?
The answer that comes is "She knows."

Let me ask you, why were you shown this lifetime?
I don't know yet. (Laughs)

Hal, what's the connection between that past life and the present life?
I hear the same thing; "She knows. She knows."

Let's reach into the deepest part of you that knows the reason for that life to come forward. There could have been dozens of others, but this was the one to come forth. What's the connection between that life and now? Why were we shown that life today? What comes into your mind?
The name; June.

What would June like to give to you as a gift?
What comes to my mind is "love."

Go ahead and do that, feel the love coming from June. And if you could give June a gift, what would it be?
Strength.

Do that now, give her strength. I want to ask June, what is it that you want her to examine during this session?
She's not alone. I don't know if I have the words, but I understand that maybe she is with me now.

June had a mesmerizing experience in her life.
Yeah; she saw the eyes of Jesus.

What does that mean for your life today?
Interesting that I gave her what I thought she needed was the strength, but she might have had more than me. June.

Let's ask Hal if it has any meaningful message for you.
Oh God, what comes to mind is "What do you think?" He's a very tricky guide, he puts it right back on me.

Is there anything about the experience of Jesus that you can bring forward into your life today?
Oh, I live in that life every day. And I, you know, in my everyday life I try to be as good and kind and generous as anybody could be, I feel I'm already doing that in my life, but maybe I need to do it more.

Do you feel that looking at this life as June can energize that Jesus part of you?
Yes.

Is there something you Hal would like to guide or show us today?
I hear the same thing he's told me before when I'd be in a frenzy; "Honey if you only knew, you were already there." I hear that again now, I don't know how to interpret it, but this is what's coming to my mind.

What are you sensing right now?
"Hee hee" He's laughing. Amazing sense of humor.

You've got one of those spirit guides with a great sense of humor. All right, as we leave the realm of the soul, remember this loving worlds is always with you.. (talks her back to consciousness).

Oddly enough, a few days prior to this session, Scott and I had been speaking about how Paul Aurand, interviewed earlier in the book, had clients who lived at the time of Jesus, and I'd asked him if they could describe what he looked like. Paul said it hadn't occurred to him to ask. And now, three days later, my friend Molly remembers in vivid detail a lifetime where she had a chance to see Jesus speak and could describe how he looked. What are the odds of that?

I was equally moved to hear her account, especially being a friend who was suffering emotionally. Before the session, I warned her there was no guarantee of any past life memory at all, or a chance to speak to her departed mother. She got to do both. She was too exhausted to enter the "between lives" realm to see why she made these life choices; she opted to do that at a later date. Perhaps Scott can ask more questions about her lifetime where she saw Jesus speak. But she told me she's feeling stronger and better by just experiencing the session, and can clearly see the face of Jesus when she recalls it.

I include this chapter not as proof or evidence of any concept. Certainly, experiencing a past life memory etches it in your mind so that you feel you always have access to it, and whether it happened or not, people come away feeling as if it *was* authentic. Those who see loved ones, as Molly did, feel truly as if they're in the presence of their beloved departed ones and are comforted by knowing they still exist. But it's equally true that once someone has a strong between life memory it's etched in their minds and hearts forever.

Afterwards, Scott and I talked about the phenomenon of people like Jesus being on Earth. Obviously she was deeply moved by his presence, but I couldn't help but note the Romans were less so. My theory in this area is that Jesus showed up on Earth with a much higher percentage of his spirit than people normally do, hence why he was associated with miracles of the spirit. Those who were prepared to hear his message were deeply moved by him. Perhaps that offers some explanation of the power religious icons like Buddha, Mohammed and other religious avatars generate when they bring a message of universal and eternal love and a vision of bliss to the planet.

I like your Christ, I do not like your Christians. Your Christians are so unlike your Christ.

- Mahatma Gandhi

CHAPTER 21
BE THERE NOW

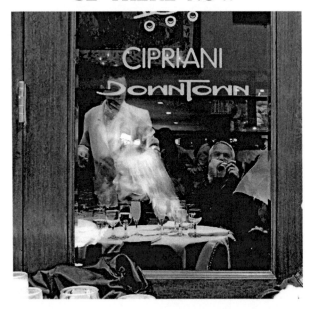

"I define synchronicity as a psychically conditioned relativity of time and space. It reveals the meaning connections between the subjective and objective world… This principle suggests that there is an inter-connection or unity of causally unrelated events, and thus postulates a unitary aspect of being which can very well be described as the "unus mundus" (One World.)"

- Carl Jung

A couple of years after my session with Jimmy, I was offered to do another Life between Lives session, with a different hypnotherapist, to see if the results were the same. The very gifted Newton trained Scott De Tamble offered to do a follow up session with me.

Me and *Scott De Tamble*

(Sessions begins with Scott walking Richard through his life. Going back to 13, 12, 11...)

Scott: Let's drift and float to the front of your home at age 11 now. Is it light or dark?
Me: Light. There's a driveway, car port and we're putting on a play - got the neighborhood kids together, there's a Chicago TV celebrity who lives up the block, Ray Rayner,[100] and his daughter Chris and I are friends, and we put on *The Sound of Music*. My first foray into show biz, but we didn't charge admission. Story of my life; giving a free show.

Let's go back to an earlier time. Let's move to age 6 doing something fun.
We're playing "Kick the Can." I can hear the cicadas whining in the trees and the sun is going down, the echoes of kids' voices as we run around these wooded areas.

Ok... so let's move back to that stairway. Down, younger and younger... before birth in the womb. As you drift and float... How do you feel?
Comfortable, my mother's a happy person; very blissful. I feel like I've chosen well, everything's going to work out.

How do you know that?
I feel very confident about my choice here. Like a very natural selection, and I'm very comfortable melding my energy with me. And then there's Mom's energy; it's a very happy energy; I'm in comfortable place - safe.

What about the brain... Are you comfortable with this brain?
Confident of everything working out, it's a happy marriage. I'll be able to do a bunch of stuff.

What sort of stuff?
The journey – the stuff I've decided I've come here to do.
    NOTE: Despite this being a marathon session between myself and Scott de Tamble, it flew by while it was occurring. I was also unusually aware during the entire session, as if I'd never left the previous session, which occurred two years prior to this one. I also had the profound sense that I was speaking as if already in the life between lives, and directing my consciousness to the various places Scott directed me.

---

[100] Ray put me on "Bozo's Circus" in 1965. My first on camera experience was freezing when Mr. Ned asked me my name. "Dick" I said, staring at the shrinking iris on the lens as it zoomed up to my face. Years later, I was lucky enough to cast Ray as a newscaster in my feature film "Limit Up." He passed away a few days after my father did - they'd stayed lifelong friends.

WHY I CHOSE THIS LIFETIME

Any ideas what they are yet?
I've chosen Richard because he's capable of doing these things I want to do. Getting him there is going to be an interesting trip, but that's the idea.

Tell me about the things you want to do.
Why did I choose Richard? Because he's going to have the capacity to have humor as well as compassion, he has a demeanor that puts him in places where he can affect events so they have a benefit for people. As a filmmaker, as a musician, just as a persona. The adventure he's on is the adventure I was aware was going to happen; that's why I chose him. Also because I have a better capacity to be more of my "self" in him, whereas in other lifetimes I didn't have that creative capacity. Do you understand what I'm saying?

Mm-hmm.
As an American Indian, you're constricted by society and mores, but the era Richard's in now almost mirrors between lives. There's complete structure and yet no structure because of free will. You can make up your structure as you want it to be through your own manipulation. And the era Richard's in now, you don't have to follow certain rules anymore, because society has shifted.

There's a freedom of creativity and activity.
If you choose a life's path, there's very few restrictions prescribed to that path. For example if you choose to be a Priest in this lifetime, there's tons of prescribed behavior that is stuck in centuries-old tradition; very difficult to break out of that. But if you choose a life of, let's say, a filmmaker or musician, you're completely at your own ability to take that wherever you want it to go. No one to inhibit you.

So this life is an opportunity for creative self-expression?
I chose him because he's going to allow me - as a team, let's say - to accomplish things that have to do with helping other individuals or changing energy patterns of other people so they can appreciate life from a different angle. That was the task when I made this life choice to be Richard, I knew he was in a time and place where we could do a lot of stuff together that would be a lot of fun, and at the same time accomplish this mission I chose to embark upon. It's been having its fits and starts of success, but you know, that always goes with the territory of trying to learn things.

Tell me more about the mission.
Using your abilities to create things through language and film and words and music to alter other people's energy patterns to help them get to a place that's happier or more compassionate -- a place where they feel more fulfilled. By making

films or creating stories or passing information about "between lives" work; *that* helps people to understand the between lives, helps them with their present life to be in a happier place. That's always been the plan; to get him in that arena, it's taken a while; slowly but surely nudging him along.

Anything else you happen to notice about this early time before birth?
Everything fit in a nice way; I chose a lifetime and a group of people that would really nourish me. The usual amount of fears and trepidations and difficulties that come with birth and family weren't really present. I can see specific things about the journey, the visuals of what that looked like back in the 50's, that era - they're interesting people, this woman and this man[101] - she's the piano player and he's the architect; it's unusual to find people like them; happy.

Happy and creative.
Creative and artistic... Forgiving.

So this is perfect for your sort of mission.
Of course I went through the usual amount of familial stuff where your brothers don't want to let you do anything they do; but that's also character building and builds insight because it's such an important thing to instill in a human; the compassionate instinct.

From an early age, Richard would interrupt violence, or people having difficulty. Putting himself between them to calm them down or change their energy pattern; he instinctively knows how to calm people down. I'm just saying it's part of the reason I chose him.

Is this something you're interested in as a soul? Changing energy patterns?
As I've always foreseen it -- to be a healing, helpful person or a helpful, healing person -- where you use energy to change people's paradigm (i.e. primary pattern). Through medicine, healing, a spiritual endeavor; sometimes preaching... These have all been part of my journey. This time, I found somebody who could embody a little bit of all that stuff, maybe not completely to his liking... But he does have those abilities.

So you've used these modalities in different lifetimes?
Preaching, Medicine man, Doctor; I also get a sense that I was a nun as well as a spiritual path... All concern the manipulation of energy towards people to help them on their path.

NOTE: I've studied Buddhism, traveled to Dharamsala and India and made a film about Tibetan refugees. I also have traveled to Tibet with Professor Robert Thurman, as mentioned, and am familiar with the various sites that I mention in these sessions. One could argue that my having visited these monasteries and sites

---

[101] Referring to my parents Charles the architect, and Ann the concert pianist.

231

inspired my memory of them. However, I had the profound sense of returning to India and Tibet, as well as the profound sense during this session that I was viewing a movie of a previous life that I had lived.

MY LIFE AS A TIBETAN MONK

Wonderful. Let's go ahead and let go of this now, disengage and release the body and float up.. Move backward in time... To a previous incarnation... Be there now. Is it daytime or nighttime?
Night. I'm inside. I'm a Tibetan monk. I'm in the monastery, a Gompa (A Tibetan monastery). I'm barefoot I can feel the hard sandy dirt. There's a library here, but the Tibetan kind of library where the books are long and thin and kind of dusty, in candle light. The books are an odd combination of scroll and when you lift them up, each page is like a poem. These are Buddhist texts of great import. And I'm wearing an old red robe. I can feel it around me. It's cold here. I'm always cold. (I can see myself walking around with a candle.)

How long is the robe?
The robe goes all the way to the ground. It's an elaborate fold that covers your shoulders, and comes around. I want to say the year is 1650. I'm walking around where the library is, I like coming here because I enjoy reading the books by candlelight, and it's a view into the outside world. Some of the books came from India. I'm irritated by one of my teachers; the Lama in charge of our group is not very bright, and when I sit in a class with him, it annoys me because he doesn't know what he's talking about, and there's nothing I can do or say to contradict him.

He's in charge.
Because you can't contradict the teacher. I mean it's good discipline to learn in this fashion, very strict learning, but not a lot of freedom of expression here.

About how old are you?
I'm in my 30's. My name begins with N and ends in la... Nam-la. Nam is short for something.

You're in your early 30's? How do you spend your days?
It's a pretty difficult life, everyone has prescribed duties -- one day a week you might be in charge of cooking, using huge pots where all the food is cooked... Interesting, I'm seeing my friend Paul Tracey[102] here, and there's activities and there's debate every day. We do hours of debate, sometimes four hours a day where we debate the nature of existence, the nature of reality or the nature of things.

---

[102] Paul and I grew up in Northbrook together. He passed away in 2003, and is mentioned in my travels around Mt. Kailash earlier in the book.

Some of it seems very esoteric, most people don't know what they're talking about, but it's a really powerful insight into a peerless philosophy that was expounded upon by Buddha. So the actual education in the books is brilliant, but what's been espoused in this era -- there's a lot of politics involved; who's married to whom, who's related to who, and whose child did this; to me that's all nonsense.

Step outside of Namla, and describe him.
His appearance? Dirt! Mostly dirt. (Laughs) No, he's got brown hair, and Indian eyes, hooded, kind of Mongolian look, nice little ears, full lips, brown deep brown eyes, very sad look on his face, but a fun guy, funny. He's got a great sense of humor. I see a couple of scars on him as well.

On his face?
Yeah, not ugly scars, just marks. Related to... his father... as a young boy hit him for some misdeed. And his brother is a monk as well.

Let's go back to his childhood. Tell me about your father and mother.
Really harsh existence; farmers. Mother died in childbirth and father had to raise two boys, and it was just a lot of work and very difficult for him. Also trying to get a place. Not far from the Potala palace.[103] It's Sonam.

What's Sonam?
My name. Namla would be short for Sonam. I think we're a day's ride from the capital Lhasa. Where the Potala palace is. Days ride on a donkey or a horse. Mostly I walk.

Tell me about the home you share with your father.
A thatched roof kind of place further out from the city. Rudimentary. I see, this (My life as a monk) was a negotiation... Very common where a farmer, a poor family, will donate their son to the monastery in return for their protection, so when there's a famine or something the monastery takes care of the people, if there are food shortages, and there are quite a few, they'll get a ration of food. I think I was the first one to go in the monastery and then my little brother came to join me.

What's his name?
Begins with a T... Tashi, that's it... He's a playful kid.

What are the walls made of?
Mud and straw, there are quite a few homes made out of stucco or plaster water and stuff. But dad was really a poor farmer.

---

[103] The Potala Palace is in Lhasa, Tibet, and was the seat of the Dalai Lamas. I've been there and shot my film "Journey Into Tibet" there, so none of these images or names are unfamiliar to my conscious self.

What kind animals does he have?
Goats. We don't have that many. The death of his wife was a big blow. I was about six. I don't remember her very well, it affected him, and I went into the monastery not long after. He saw that it was going to be difficult. So this was a way - he was going to take care of one boy and donate the other to the monastery, a very common thing -- every family donates one child. It's just how things are done.

So that's how this child is taken care of and fed.
And taught. The only way for real education is to go to the monastery. You can choose to leave the monastery later, you can quit if you choose to, "no harm no foul," but you lose the protectorship of the monastery in case of calamity.

But the educational part of it is what I like, because it's opening up the world. Such a meager existence, and then to step into a library and find out the mysteries of the Universe… It's really unusual.

So let's go back to your life in the monastery. Tell me about the place where you sleep.
(I saw in my mind's eye a small dark room) It's a cell, a very small room. I've earned this room as librarian - you begin sleeping with everyone else, with all these people in a room, but at some point you get your own little hovel where you can do your prayers and meditations. And this is a place that has blankets and I sleep there, meditate there, go through the various tantric meditations monks do.

At least you have your own space.
It's not really in our consciousness to have your own stuff, because everything is a gift. The whole concept as a monk - your clothes are donated, your food is donated, everything is donated, and as soon as you try to attach… when you try to attach yourself to items and things, it sends you down this path of defeat. You mentally say "Well this is the place I'm in and it's as good as any other, and if allows me to have some solitude I can focus on my meditations, so that's a value." Plus in my case it's just good to get away from that stupid teacher. My little spot.

Tell me about being a librarian.
Cataloguing, putting books up, in order of the person who wrote it and their importance in the pantheon of Tibetan studies. There are books about Naropa and Tilopa and Atisha, and I have all these names on the tip of my tongue, but they're pandits from India from the 600's on up and they taught various yogas, and the higher lamas perfect these yogas and can do extraordinary things of wonder.

The library work is just keeping it organized, books dusted and when somebody needs a text, I'm the one who tracks it down and delivers it to the monk. When he's done I clean it up, make sure everything is in place, because the pages get mixed up -- really annoying... I'm trying to picture where this is…

Is it in a town?
I'm pretty sure it's behind Lhasa, which is the Capital. A day's ride away. Might be Ganden... There are big schools, but this isn't one of them, this is somewhere in between those.

So in this monastery you mentioned Paul Tracey. Is he there?
I saw him as my brother, now a monk - Tashi… Tashi = Tracey. Same name! And he's very well liked, he's a handsome fellow and very bright, very happy... Not a good student, but he makes up for it with his pure energy. I mean he doesn't care much about the deeper studies. I'm a little bit more into the deeper studies, he's more invested in the things of the world let's say; more attached.

NOTE: Before attending a session, it's customary to bring a list of friends you might encounter along the journey. As mentioned throughout this book, Paul has shown up in various places in my life since I first met him in seventh grade. I've always considered him a spiritual brother, and he was treated as if he was my brother during his albeit short lifetime.

DINING IN TIBET

Let's go to a time forward or back as Sonam. When you're having a meal; just be there.
We always dine together. It's a huge crowd of us, big communal meal, these big copper pots filled with rice. Or soup and vegetables and a myriad of spices because everything in this altitude is sort of tasteless and if you really work hard you can get interesting flavors out of it, but generally... It's part of your daily meditation to be focused on other things while you're doing something, so you don't spend a lot of time savoring, you spend time thinking about other deep thoughts while you're dining... It's kind of funny, "Why not just enjoy the soup?"

Let's go to a time when you're bathing.
Bathing? Nobody bathes here, are you kidding? Bathing is suicide. You go stand in a creek; as you step out, you'd turn to ice. The dirt becomes a protective layer of skin. Oddly enough, not my habit, but some people actually paint themselves with this thick goo and their faces turn red and it protects them from the brightness of the sun, but when you come upon them they're really scary looking painted people.

But in terms of cleanliness, you use a bowl of warm water which is put outside your door by a monk's assistant, it's hot water, sometimes a strong detergent, but to actually get into a bathtub - that's really only for the highest people. (To bathe) you just go out in the lakes; there are beautiful, the most amazing, lakes in Tibet and swimming in them is like swimming in ice water, but it's great, fabulous. I'm laughing to myself because Richard actually dunked himself in a Tibetan lake.[104] He re-lived the coldness of Tibetan water.

Go to a proud moment in the life of Sonam... Namla...
It's interesting to look for pride because you're not supposed to be proud. I earned a teaching degree - you've gone through your monastery classes and all your debates and you win your debate, which I did, by crushing the opponent with clever logistics of language.

Is there a ceremony?
Everyone is there, two or three thousand monks lined up, it's a series of tests that go on for a week, you have all kinds of exams, you have to show your ability to do "mudra" which is a kind of dance that you do with your hands, there's dancing. The most interesting are the educational games where you show your prowess with words and logic and the ability to argue a point - it might even be as silly as "Is white a color or the absence of color?[105]" where one person takes one side and the other monks take the other side. Mine were always arguments about examining the nature of reality. And I (see that I) have a teacher who gets me, who understands me. Not the guy who was in my classes that I was so annoyed by, but somebody who's a higher lama who appreciated my arguments. He's a visiting judge and was able to award us the Geshe[106] title, Geshe which means teacher, it's a big deal, there's a buzz about it. Geshe-la.

How many monks are awarded this?
About 20 at the moment; people who've gone through all their monastic studies.

Let's go to an important moment in your life, a turning point...
It's... my health. I'm old... about 86, I've got this cough that's not leaving. I'm on my way, on the journey, on the path - not something I'm particularly afraid of, it's just annoying to have to cough, and then when you get a death rattle in these places, you echo everywhere, the sound of coughing and your attendant trying to come and help you.

So you got a pretty bad cough.
It's pneumonia. Not much longer for this world. It's now about 1710. Trying to see if I can pinpoint which Dalai Lama is in residence... I think it's the 7th.[107]

---

[104] While circling Mt. Kailash with Robert Thurman I took the opportunity to dunk myself in sacred Lake Mansarovar. Oddly enough, I heard my father's voice say loudly "That's enough!" and I got out of the freezing water before I froze any further.

[105] While visiting Dharamsala in 1997, I asked Professor Thurman to describe a typical debate issue, he said "It might be as simple as "Is white a color?" So, I was familiar with this concept.

[106] "Teacher" in Tibetan. It's an honorific title given to those who've graduated certain Buddhist classes.

[107] The 7th Dalai Lama was from 1708–1757

Let's move to the last day... Of Sonam.
I'm falling over; I was in an equipoise position, it's early in the morning about 3:30 in the morning and it's before my attendant has come to find me. I'm standing up and looking down at myself as this old monk. Who is no longer on the planet.

How do you feel about the life you just left?
I'm reflecting on the lessons I learned, and I'm cherishing the connections with other monks and friends. I have relationships with other lamas in the kind of position I'm in, where you're teasing them. Only they can laugh at it, because others don't get the humor. I'm seeing another old monk. He'll be one of the few people who mourn my passing. At this point I'm just an old lama somebody's taking care of. Everybody I knew is gone, most of them didn't make it this far.

No sadness, just a reflection on how I chose to be this monk, chose to experience this world from that point of view, and surprisingly didn't have any kind of extreme tragedy happen. I seem pretty content.

Is there anything you need to do before you go?
I'll stop by my attendant's room and blow out the candles to let him know I've passed. That wakes him up. My little sense of humor. I feel myself patting him on the head. Young kid. Thanking him for his service. Okay, I'm good to go.

NOTE: I saw this all clearly and experienced these events as if they'd happened to me. I could feel the rattle in my throat as I mentioned it, as well as feel the affection that I had for what I reported was my attendant. I could feel the cold from the monastery, and could sense that death was imminent. I also saw the flickering candles as I blew them out.

A JOURNEY BACK

Okay, now you're flying into deep space. How does that feel?
Liberating. Just liberating. I've done this journey before -- It's that journey of complete release and returning home, almost like a magnet pulling you back. I feel like I'm moving so quickly, so rapidly it's not as if I'm pulling myself or forcing myself through space, but the opposite - the way a magnet pulls a piece of filament across the table.

Like you're whooshing back.
Like your whooshing back with all your loved ones. I'm looking for my spirit guide.

Just give yourself time to relax and release.
If it makes any sense I'm getting the feeling that Rayma, my spirit guide -- he's advising me there's another lifetime they want me to examine. Before coming back here.

So let's go ahead and do that.
It's just this feeling the brakes are on; "Turn around." Let's go back, let's examine. This American Indian fellow again. I'm sorry, it's India. Not Indian. A journey to Bombay.

NOTE: When I landed at the airport in Bombay for the first time, I had the profound sense that I was returning to India. I spent time in Kerala, and visited the home of a higher caste family that was involved with decorating elephants in gold during the Ahrjatpuram festival held in Thrichur. So when I describe the following places and events, I had a basis already in my head for the visuals I described. However, like the other lifetimes I examined, they all felt as if they were memories from my own life.

LIFETIME AS A BRAHMIN PRIEST

Let's follow his guidance, and follow the feeling.
Okay, it's another Priest. This one is a Brahmin Priest. Somebody darker skinned. Another form of religious persecution, where you're born into this group and they teach you these mysteries of the Universe, and there's a huge amount of laws and regulations and dictates about the way people should walk and talk and what squiggle on their forehead is important. I'm married, I've got two children.

Tell me about your wife.
She's dark, black eyes, black hair, very beautiful. She's short, sweet spirit, I married her because of her smile. We're a higher caste so we live in a nicer area, a house with many rooms; there's a fountain in the center like Kerala[108], they've got beds that hang from the ceiling, so when you climb into bed you're always rocking, always moving subtly, it's nice.

There are religious regulations you have to learn and memorize; protocol and caste and who's who in the zoo, but I get a sense I'm just anti all that stuff. I'm considered a holy man, because I greet anybody in the street anywhere; give the same amount of time, the same kind of dedication or kindness.

Your wife?
Her name is Miriam. My name means holy man. She says it teasingly. It's Sam... something.

What's the work you do?
There's the temple and inside the temple is the holy of holies and inside the holy of holies is a holy book or a garment that is kept. This is sacred because it has to do with the Bhagavad-Gita (a sacred Hindu philosophical text). In this case it's a rock;

---

[108] I've been to Kerala, and seen large homes with baths in the center, as well as beds that hang on swings, so what I speak of isn't new to me. I've also seen a Brahmin temple in Kerala.

interesting, it's a rock from Mt. Kailash[109] where Krishna was born.

I have friends I chat with and intellectuals that come to me to seek out knowledge. And we talk about the mysteries of the Universe and my own esoteric ideas of how the planet works and they bring alms and all kinds of gifts. It's something you have to protect against, because they want to buy influence from the Priest, gold is the big commodity, so people press it on me all the time. I see it as a way of attachment, so I put that stuff away mostly.

Why are we here seeing this life?
I'm here to see my spiritual connection to India. It runs deep since Richard was a child. He wrote papers about India,[110] had a pen pal in India[111], and he's been to many places in India. But it reminds him of what he doesn't like about India - the caste concept. Why should somebody born with darker color skin have to suffer immeasurably, versus me, who's got like this almost bronze colored skin, a genetic flaw that was passed along in the Brahmin culture?

It's a fascinating place, there are other religious leaders here, and from Buddhists I meet, to Parsi (a Persian religion the migrated to India in the 10th century). It's a time of sacred things where everything has an energy to it that's sacred, a time of honoring that sacred energy. It's also a time of intense plagues and people dying, "Why did this happen to me?" and I try not to say "It's God's will;" or "It's Brahma." I try not to go down that path...

I'm trying to see what the markings are on my forehead because that dictates who I am... I see a white line like a river, there's three of them - ok, that's the sect that I belong to, Krishna's sect. There are three, river-like; they go down,[112] some people have it across, each one represents a story in the Bhagavad-Gita, as it tells people on the street instantly what it is you're a preacher of.

So three white lines down your forehead?
They waver like water. You put them on each day, there's a little holy kit that has Aruveydic makeup with its healing qualities. A lot of ritual involved. When you're talking about things that are sacred you spend a lot of time paying homage to the sacredness of these things, and ignore the hypocrisy outside the door. As if to say "Here I am applying this makeup; meanwhile a guy down the block is starving.

---

[109] Mt. Kailash is sacred to the ancient Tibetan Bon, the Jain, the Hindu and Buddhism.

[110] My first researched paper in grade school was on India and its independence, probably influenced by having a pen pal from Kerala.

[111] The pen pal was from Thrichur, and oddly enough, I shot footage of her hometown, but wasn't there long enough to find her. Her local Priest, Father Matthew Kalalakal, had come to visit my home in Northbrook, and suggested the pen pal program.

[112] In India, a Brahman is a member of the priestly caste of India, they paint three horizontal lines or a vertical trident on their foreheads. From a website on Hindu markings: "They are of two kinds—the trident shaped mark called urdhva pundram or upright pun-dram, worn by the votaries of Vishnu, and the three horizontal lines drawn across the forehead, called tiryak pundram or horizontal pundram, worn by the worshippers of Siva." I didn't know these details until I looked them up on the internet post LBL.

Wouldn't it make sense to just go help him?" That's just my sense of humor.

So this lifetime as Sam.
It's a longer name like Samvarta. Let's just call him Sam.

What does Sam's life have to do with Richard's life?
Every one of these lives has to do with energy transformation, and in that time and era, whether as a Healer or Priest, it's about the journey of energy and trying to connect to sacred energy, which is another way to put it. What Richard doesn't have in his vocabulary yet is that Energy is sacred. There's such a thing as Sacred Energy -- another way to look at this kind of work. If you consider it sacred, you behave around it in a different fashion. In the positive term of Sacred which is to pay homage to it - to take more care with it, to be more careful about it. It also relates to your work (Scott's hypnotherapy work) as well. You're dealing with sacred things and the work pays homage to the sacredness of it. It's a way to connect to the Divine, using the word Divine to mean "the blissful all-powerful nature of the Universe." I don't really want to use that word, but that's the definition of The Divine.

AN INTERVIEW WITH MY SPIRIT GUIDE

Let me ask your guide's advice, shall we use this Indian life to transition to the LBL?
It's as if we're speaking from the life between lives already, we don't really need to take the journey per se, because we're already there. I don't know why that is, but it seems like whatever this session is about, we're skipping down to what needs to be said.

Let's ask your guide what to call him for this session.
Rayma.

Let's take him to an LBL spot where you can sit and talk.
We're in a beautiful field, under a tall oak tree. There's a pretty river nearby; it's a place we've been before, grass growing, slight wind in the air; sunshine.

What's your guide saying?
(Laughs) "What is it you want to know? What's up?"

Rayma, gives us a name for Richard's soul here. What's his soul name?
For the sake of this session, let's call him Richard.

What's Richard's first life memory?
(Speaking in a different tone as spirit guide Rayma) First life memory on Earth was in Mesopotamia, Iraq, 5 to 6000 years ago, a simple life as a boy/farmer. I say boy because he didn't live long. (He was here) just to get a taste of what Earth is like, all of the sensations and tastes, flavors, and he did a lot before he died at 13. He

died in a stone quarry, killed by stones. His first life was wonderful as he was able to get a sense of connections to people; mother, father, sisters and brother. Family connections.

On a non-Earth material plane? First lifetime?
As in previous to lifetimes on Earth? Yes. There was one on a planet in another galaxy, a beautiful setting with a forest. The creatures are simple organisms, not very complex and he had a life there. Of course I was with him then, as we were just starting out life together.

It's part of my plan for this guy (Richard). We've been working on it for millennia. Part of my agreement to be his life guide so we would go on this journey together and I'd do my best to help him master these things, a lot of them have to do with energy transfer. I was there at his birth as a soul entity, and with him ever since, 6 or 8 lifetimes before his first lifetime on Earth.

Why did you choose this other place?
This is a master journey, I'm like a painter. Let's say in my agreement and my soul journey, I take this paint - which is a soul - and map out, "What's the canvas going to be?" and "What colors are going to get the right effect?" I know it sounds egotistical, but it's an apt description of the journey.

You're kind of the artist, helping this soul.
Everyone who does this kind of work has their own method, which comes from their own experience, and in my case, I felt to get the end result, for Richard to eventually become a spirit guide and to be doing the same work I do.

NOTE: Upon reviewing the footage from this session, I confirmed what I'd felt at the time I was speaking; the words came through me like chunks of paragraphs being spit out of a teletype machine. I spoke rapidly without taking a breath, and it took me several attempts to transcribe the paragraphs I was speaking in, as if I was trying to get as much information out as possible. If one reads the words at double speed, that's about how fast I was saying them.

HOW A SPIRIT GUIDE IS CREATED

And Richard's destiny is to be a teacher/guide like you?
That's everyone's basic journey. Everyone's spirit guide helps lead them through these many lifetimes so they get to a point where they can do the same. Then turn and give the same gift for other souls. In Richard's case, we started off in simplistic settings, I won't go into detail, but they were places like a gymnasium where a spirit works out the details. By the time we decided to go to Mesopotamia, I want to say 6 or 7000 years ago, he was 'ready to go' -- to go and sense and see. And Earth is so rich with its experiences, much deeper and richer than these other places.

You did a warm-up. So why Earth?
Earth is *the* playground. It's the ballgame, whereas other places are like being in the parking lot outside the stadium. And once you get into the Earth game, it's really a wonderful, terrific place to come and do these experiences. The Earth realm mimics the life between life realm in many ways. You have all these same souls doing the same kind of work, same kind of journey they do in the between-worlds. So this ball game, let's call it that because there's violence that happens, and there's a lot of activity running around in circles ostensibly, but that kind of journey mimics the spirit world. And you can spiritually progress by going through intense experiences here when you might not progress over there (raises hand to indicate another world) It might take you 5,000 years over there to learn what you can learn here in a day, going through an incredible tragedy. Does that make sense?

THE STADIUM KNOWN AS EARTH

So the point of incarnating on Earth is to accelerate learning?
To accelerate the experience of a spiritual journey - accelerate is not the right word, but "to experience in a deeper, richer fashion." You certainly can experience those things by observation - like when you sit in a theater and watch a play; you can experience loss and pain and tragedy from your seat. Doing it yourself, as you can imagine, is much richer, almost like the engrams[113] of your energy system experience it in a deeper fashion when it's first hand.

But that being said, there are people who say "No thanks, I'm going to watch from the stadium, I'm not going into the gladiator pit, I don't have to be pilloried in order to experience that." And they're right, you don't have to be, you can sit up there and experience it. If you're the kind of individual who needs that kind of passionate jumpstart, or wants it -- there are people like that; who want to dive into the deep end of the pool. And there's nothing wrong with that; to be a warrior who dives in feet first and really wants to get a bath by fire. Earth is a place where you can do it. There's such capacity here, because there's so many souls here.

These other places where people incarnate are like vacation spots. You get a loofa scrub (laughs) on your soul. You float through that life, sort of getting your toenails done and maybe one or two annoying thing happens, but you experiencing things at a slower pace, even while you are progressing spirituality. They don't have the intensity of Earth.

A LIFETIME AS A DOCTOR IN BOSTON

A question from his list. Was he a doctor in Boston?
Yes. Civil War was happening in the US, but his political bent was anti-slavery, an abolitionist in Boston in the 1860's, I want to say Shelby is his name. He's a doctor,

---
[113] Engram; a hypothetical means by which memory traces are stored. Wikipedia. (A word I had to look up later)

lives on Beacon Hill, and has a fairly successful practice, beautiful home - first name... Marian. Marian or Martin Shelby.[114]

What about his family?
His wife is (his current wife) Sherry, he's got four children, two girls and two boys. Very easy going, another easy life for this guy because we know how to pick 'em. A Doctor with all the medical practice of that era, the nonsense of the old-fashioned ways.

What did he gain?
When you're a Doctor you're always manipulating energy, and you're connecting to the energy of the Universe, whether you know it or not. As a healer, doing it through surgery or through energetic movement, it's all the same energy and the same methods. The first time you help or cure someone, your life changes; you've saved a life, you've cured somebody. You're not really sure why it worked, but it puts you in the mindset of continuing to do that.

But there's a sadness in this life. I think it has to do with that he had bigger dreams for himself. Like a higher calling he thought he had, but because of the Brahmin society of the era, which is funny; he was a Brahmin in one life in India, and a Brahmin in this life in Boston as they're known.

What was he aspiring to?
He was a Doctor in a Catholic Boston hospital[115] and defeated by the politics within. He wanted to help the impoverished people of the North End, the Italians and Poles and Portuguese, but the hospital wouldn't allow it. And it depressed him, defeated him. He was happy at home, I see a happy guy, kind of overweight, watch fob, vest, white curly hair, moustache, sad eyes.

NOTE: Sometime after this session, I was at an antique store and saw a wooden Doctor's drug case. I've no recollection of seeing one before, but recognized what it was. I also had a quick flash of dread seeing it, visualizing injecting myself with a brass needle of some drug. Perhaps medicine, or addicted to something in the kit.

HOW TO CHANNEL HEALING ENERGY

Let's go to the Lakota Sioux medicine man lifetime...
His name was Wa'tanka,[116] "Man of Great Spirit." The American Indian people are very connected to the life between lives world, which they refer to as "The Great Spirit." Both the American Indians and the aboriginal tribes of Australia

---

[114] Marian Shelby appears in indexes in the late 1800's in the South. Dr. Shelby practiced in Missouri in the late 1800's.

[115] In Boston, Catholic hospitals included St. Elizabeth's Hospital (1868), the Free Home for Consumptives 1891, the Holy Ghost Hospital for Incurables 1893.

[116] "Sacred force, the spirit which moves in all things." Sitting Bull was known as "Tatanka Watanka"

have much to offer (with their knowledge); it's amazing so few on the planet have focused on their wisdom (with regard to the spirit world and nature).

As a medicine man, people would bring him their sick and he would pray over them and would use the equivalent to calling upon the Great Spirit to heal them. When you put your mindset into that frame, whatever culture you're from, you tap into that healing energy of the universe -- which is facilitated through you, through your hands and into the patient, and depending upon their karmic journey, let's call it that for want of a better word; they get healed. So if you're good at it, you can affect a lot of lives.

Richard has asked for details.
That's something Richard is aware of - in the Tibetan culture there's a healing meditation called "Tonglen,"[117] it's effective. It's a practice he's studied before, and he should tell people about it. Most consider prayer to be of the same system, but there are certain techniques you can use to perfect, train the mind, so it can help focus that healing energy.

Give us a one, two, three recipe on how to do this.
First the mind should go through a gymnastic period. Picture your patient in 360 degrees, as a vision of a three dimensional character, sitting in front of you, then imagine where the illness is - that's a way of doing gymnastics for your own mind and it also benefits the patient. Tune your mind to the patient, 2nd, put the patient in front of you as a mental image because you're replicating their energy, and 3rd then alter their energy or focus on healing them.

One example would be someone with pneumonia, or chest pain. Picture that person in an energetic pattern in front of you, what's bothering them will have a different color to it, a different glow - and then this Tibetan exercise is effective, you draw that energy into you, pull the illness into you, and use your ability to tap into the healing light of the universe to dissolve that negativity, and then breathe the transformed healing light back into the patient.

NOTE: Scott took the opportunity to ask questions that he was curious about.

PARALLEL LIVES

Can people have parallel lives? Or lives that overlap?
It depends on the person. There are people that can have parallel lives, meaning their energy is in two people simultaneously. If everyone has 100% energy in the afterlife, let's say only 50% comes to Earth, and you split out the other 25% and another 25% into other human beings... do the math. It's a rare thing to do, a complicated maneuver and only really adept souls can try to pull it off.

---

[117] Tibetan for "giving and taking"

What are the major lessons he learned in the Sioux Indian lifetime?

Learning the healing energy; the major thing he went through was as a healer of his people. Then there's the Sioux connection to the planet, awareness of the Earth in terms of finding it sacred. All native cultures honor the Earth in that way, ironic that the non-native cultures don't – because it's paramount.

But in Richard's case, this Sioux life was important because once his family was killed, he wound up drifting. Everything was taken from him; it was important to experience that. When the things you find sacred are taken away from you, you discover nobody wants to hear you're a healer, nobody wants to be healed; you find a world of dark individuals focused on themselves. It's important to see that because then you can focus on trying to heal yourself. He gave up at some point and killed himself because his culture and his life had been turned inside out.

AN EXPLORATION OF SUICIDE

So when someone decides to check out, when they could persevere, how do you feel about that?

It's a lot of work to get to paint on the canvas - to manipulate the canvas, get all the colors on it and put them in perspective. It's a lot of work to get incarnated. All this hard work and everyone's involved and there's many spirits and souls and individuals and guides - everyone putting their best efforts -- to make this *thing* work. It's devastating to everyone when it fails.

But failure is of course a relative term; it doesn't mean "failure" per se, you're talking about a journey of a thousand lifetimes, what do you call the one or two that fizzled out? A miss-step? But all these people connected to you have put their intention towards the success of your life, and for those who succeed in overcoming a disaster, overcoming suicidal feelings, they benefit everyone and we all feel it – we're all able to embrace that victory. "You pulled it off this time, you were able to overcome it!" would be a way of putting it.

But there's no dishonor in the life between lives; it doesn't exist, there's none of it, you don't experience things from disappointment or dishonor or any *dis* - there's no diss. (Laughs) It's all honor and understanding and embracing, because you're helping. Your compassion is great to help another soul.

If you look at it from the point of view of compassion - whatever somebody else's journey is, you just completely want to be at the service of that person to do the best for themselves, and of course like any parent, like any teacher who watches a student fail - you take it upon yourself; "I screwed up. I didn't show them the path in the best way that I could have. Somehow I failed."

And then of course, your logic tells you "No, I didn't fail; it's part of their journey." It's part of the examination of life. Buddhism points to it in a way, to the idea of detachment of "value added systems" with regard to judging actions of behavior. When you judge somebody else's path, you're adding value judgment to it, where it may or may not exist for that person.

If someone does something bad, like suicide, you have a choice whether to feel sad or happy for them. On one hand, you could feel happy for them because now they're going to get to their next journey faster. If somebody commits suicide, as weird as it sounds, it's "Okay, let's pick up our tools again and let's get back to the canvas and let's find out how to do this a proper way." It's one way to look at it. And it's a way of honoring that person to say "You know what? It didn't work, we understand, we're going to find a way to help you make it work next time."

THE HEALTH OF THE PLANET

He wants advice on healthful eating.
The concept of organic food is the right path, to eat locally and organically, the more you do that, the more you avoid toxins. There's an energy factor with food, which is complicated, but worth examination; the thing you're about to eat - what was the energy pattern of it before you ate it? How did it get into this energy form? It's not that a cow gets shot and then you experience being shot, but it is on some subatomic energy level, true that many cows are tortured before being ground into your common burger. It does affect you energetically. There's all kinds of preservatives or other chemicals in water and food - it's like a mine field, it's amazing human bodies adapt to all kinds of nonsense.

PRE LIFE MEETING WITH A SOUL MATE AND CHILDREN

So did he and his wife Sherry have a pre-discussed agreement to get together?
Absolutely. It was the day he had to remember that necklace, (Sherry's necklace that she wore the day they met at Starbucks)[118] that was the clue given to him to remember. And it wasn't until he saw it, that it drew his attention -- and then he saw her, and in that moment, they had a pure examination of their energy together. And because he was already on some other path and he was charging up another hill, it took him some time to get back down the hill and to get back connected with her. She's a guardian angel who grounds him. People in your soul group are like guardian angels. -- So yes, they've been together, they've agreed to be together, their children have been with them before; they're all very connected to the life between lives in this life.

His daughter Olivia talks about being in "the angel realm." What's that?
She remembered her life between lives and called it the angel realm, and spoke of people that were in the angel realm with her. She said her brother wasn't in her realm but in the "I love you realm" - that's just a playful way to describe a neighboring soul group - the "I love you" group, the "Angel Group."

---

[118] As noted earlier, the day I met my wife, she was wearing a necklace that caught my eye.

What about the word she spoke as she was being born?[119]
Heggadaba! (Laughs) It means "I'm coming" both "out" and "back;" the same thing literally. It's more like "Here's Johnny." When you show up in a room and say "I'm here" or "I'm back" or "there you are;" same thing.

What language is that?
It's a life between lives language.

There is a language?
When people are asked "What's the name of your spirit guide?" people answer with a word so you can understand it, but it's more like a sound. "Rayma" is not really a word; it's more like "Raayyymmaazhh." More of a sound. Where did the language originate? That's beyond my scope.

Any Earth language related to this?
Well, it's another form of communication. Earth language is based on glottal stops and the way your mouth works, this language is based on no mouths, people aren't talking, they're using energy, so it's closer to like when you hear the sound of a machine, like the high pitched whine of an engine.

A musical instrument?
Absolutely, closer to instruments than language.

Richard tends to live long lives and die of old age.
It comes from very careful planning. (Laughs) You get more bang for your buck if you choose a life that doesn't have a violent ending. I mean it's hard to avoid it certainly, and a lot of people don't want to, because they want to experience that journey, but for specific reasons, Richard is manufactured in such a way as to avoid violence. He tends to not create it and tends to avoid or dissipate it. I guess you could just say he's a benevolent spirit. Hard to explain why, because there's no judgment there. It has to do with the structure of the energy when it's put together at its inception.

Was it another tribe that destroyed his tribe during his life as an American Indian?
The Huron tribe. An argument over what one Chief had said about another Chief. You know how it goes, one Chief sends out warriors over a human foible.

Where was Richard?
He was gathering medicine. He was subconsciously aware something bad was going to happen. He didn't realize it was going to be in his home, in his teepee, he thought it would be a battle between the two tribes, and was out picking up <u>medicine; herbs,</u> medicinal flowers for the coming battle, to help heal wounds he

---

[119] As mentioned previously, before Olivia emerged from her mother during birth, she opened her eyes and spoke. The Doctor looked at me as if to say "Did you hear that?"

knew would come. He returned and saw the disaster happening and instead of being caught, ran up this hillside until he got to a place of safety. His feet were all cut up and that's where he began his vision, his bloody feet in a creek. There's a certain feeling of guilt of not being there with his family and friends as they were hacked to death.

LIFETIME AS A SUMERIAN PRIEST

Let's examine other friends that Richard may have been with before...
He and Luana had a connection a long time ago.

Let's explore that.
Sumerian priests of a cult.[120] Luana and Richard. The religion is a bit like Zoroastrianism (a 6th century BC Persian religion). The same concept people have of Judaic temples, because the Jews borrowed some of that from previous religions, the Egyptians specifically; you have the Temple and you have holy people in the Temple -- nothing like it is today, absent of conflict. The Temple back then was a cacophony of people - you even had Temple sex workers there, almost like an office building with people who had various jobs. There are the money lenders - where'd you go to borrow money. If you wanted an attorney, you'd go to the temple, your odds of getting a pretty decent hooker are better than if you go to some roadside inn - There's lots of pejoratives involved, but that's where you went - that was the hub of civilization, the Temple.

NOTE: I've never heard nor researched anything about Sumeria. I may have seen the word in a museum, but have no conscious concept of where or what it is.

But if you were lucky enough to be born into a temple society - it was by birth and never by being chosen - you were able to rise through the ranks. Every now and then you'd find truly spiritual people.

Sumerian priests were more involved in animism, worshipping fire, water, air, wind, Earth...[121] But also the light and dark, that whole big bugaboo about dark spirits - that's how you keep people in line; you scare the hell out of them and they'll line up. But Luana and Richard were both Priests, but it's a deeper connection, kindred spirits. I'm getting an image of temples and candles and incense.

They both saw everything as not too serious and were playful spirits, let's put it that way. Both happy to deal with spirituality in a serious way, but they just see the value of lightness in dealing with these issues and have always been comedic spiritualists for lack of a better term.

---

[120] Sumeria: "Land of the Lords of Brightness." In Mesopotamia, 5-3000 BCE. Earliest known civilization. Each city state was centered around a Temple dedicated to a patron God or Goddess.

[121] According to Grolier Electronic Encyclopedia 1993, Sumerian key Gods were Enki (water), Ki (Earth) Enlil (Air) and An (Heaven.). According to Wikipedia, Sumerian Priests were viewed as mediums between humans and the cosmic forces.

What did Luana's last words mean? Her last words being "Ha ha ha?"[122]
She saved that up as a way of saying goodbye. A way of laughing and saying goodbye at the same time, she didn't have the breath to say it in the laughter, so she just said the words - it was also a message to focus on the comedy of life, as opposed to the seriousness of what was happening. In reflection of what I just said, that even in the most serious situation, she was so aware of her dying and the condition she was in, but laughed to remind him of the comedy of it all. If you're going to sum up a life in three words, "Ha Ha Ha," would be a clever way to do it.

What's the significance of creativity in Richard's life?
Art has its own energy, as humans do. You can't dictate what humans are going to do; you can put them in the right direction, and they may do the right thing, but then again they may screw up, or take their own life; you can put them in the right path but it's really up to them.

So the same thing is true with art; all art is emotion and all emotion is energy. Energy has its own life. And you can put all your energy into some project and it may just float off in another direction, and sometimes there's no amount of careful planning and tinkering that can alter that; art has a life of its own and you just have to honor that, chalk it up to experience. But the energy's the same if you create a magnificent pizza everyone enjoys, or you create a magnificent pizza only you eat. Or you may create it in your own mind, but the energy in the creation is the same. The value is the same. Does that make sense?

I think so.
When you create a movie or a song, even if no one hears it, the energy of creation is the same -- if everyone on the planet hears it, the energy is the same. Certainly people are influenced by it, but the end result is the same for you, that's why you need to honor even the smallest thing you put your energy into. Even the tiniest note of a symphony you're trying to create. If you make that little note sacred - you've imbued it with these wonderful qualities that will protect it as it moves through the Universe. It's ok to send it out there willy-nilly too, but you feel better when you put sacred intention into making something.

That's just the nature of art. There's no point in lamenting it, (when it fails) because it mirrors life, it mirrors the energy of life, which is that journey we take and things happen that are mysterious and unusual, no matter what the journey is.

Even in a spirit guide's journey there is learning. Even when you've become a non-reincarnating spirit you keep learning, even though you're not coming down here to Earth to learn it. You've dedicated your life - imagine that, if you will - you've dedicated your existence to this one individual's life journey. That gift is really an amazing energy transference - to keep an eye on somebody for millennia. Can you imagine? And while they go through change it affects you as well, you

---

[122] As Luana died, she turned to me and said "Ha, ha, ha" before she passed away.

learn and you experience things too, Eventually you get to that end and you've made it to a higher degree, a higher energy field and you keep going up that ladder, till you get to the top. (Laughs) I can't tell you about the top. That's not allowed. No, I mean the top is the great divine energy of the universe, you're just working your way back to that.

MESSAGES FROM A HEALER IN THE SPIRIT REALM

Are there any messages for Luana's friends?
Yes, one close friend asked Richard to tell Luana she loves her and Luana wants to say that she misses her and loves her every day - every moment - and Luana's message is; -- (pause) Luana, if you don't mind we need to hear your voice -- (pauses as if having a conversation). Any messages for your friends? Anything in particular?...

She's questioning me "What, are you on a television show?" "No, I'm not, just asking…" She's laughing, that's a joke. I say "Anything you want to tell your friends?" She says "Other than I love you eternally, forever? No." She's saying something along the lines of "The moment when you least expect it, there I am, and every moment you think of me, there I am." And "Keep up the good work." So that's her message to her friends; "Keep up the good work."

Can I ask what she's involved in right now?
She's been involved in healing energy work for a long time - dating back to when we first met and in her journey in this lifetime she chose to be an actress because she felt that she could heal and help people through her very intense acting style, she greatly influenced people around her, including close friends like Jack (Nicholson) - helping them become a complete other character; that was her gift. But all along, she knew she would never attain the kind of status and fame that her close friends did.[123]

However, the intensity she approached her art with was detrimental to her health, she knew it would be; her complete involvement in certain pained characters, and also painful things that happened to her as a youth, kept the illness hidden within her. But she was aware that was going to happen as well. Not so young perhaps, but it was part of the journey she signed up for.

In the spirit realm?
She continues to help people that are Healers, in accessing the healing light in the Universe. Very specifically she might be in alongside a doctor doing an operation, or alongside a Healer, helping channel the energy from the Universe into a patient to heal them.

I'm also getting that she's reincarnated - I want to say she's a young girl in Japan - but (as in other cases) only a certain percentage of her energy is here. (She's a)

[123] Luana's friends include multiple Academy Award winning actors, writers and directors.

very strong person, so she's helping some little girl in Japan. Which is another way of looking at reincarnation by the way - your higher self is helping some person through a journey and you gain benefit from it. She's helping this little girl in Japan right now, named Yoshi, something. She's enjoying it.

I'm confused. She's helping her? Or she's somehow shadowing her?
I'm sort of expanding the concept of reincarnation; which is that you are you, and you are also your higher self. And your higher self generally retains quite a bit of energy - it's not the way that we see it - (from the human perspective we see) that our human bodies have all our energy, it's not that way, (it's the other way around). Our higher selves retain most of our energy, so you see how it's almost like a direct link with the human to help them through their path. Does this make sense?

NOTE: Debbie Haynie echoes this: "We are spiritual beings that live on this Earth. We're not Earthly beings who happen to be spiritual, but the other way around."

PERCENTAGES OF SOUL ENERGY

So what percentage of Richard's soul energy is here?
35 percent. I'm also getting the impression it's not a finite figure, when people answer that question, answer should be "it depends." At the moment you ask the question they'll say, "I'm 35% here and 65% there." But it's not a finite number through the whole lifetime journey, because there are other moments when you have better access. I'll give you a few; a person in a coma, they're completely accessible, a person asleep...

When you say in a coma, 100% is available?
It's like they can go back and forth, because once your animal self is shut down they have total access to your higher self; you can then make the percentage one percent, or two percent - why have 40% of your energy in a coma, when you're not helping anyone, or helping yourself. That human is shut down, why not do some other things and leave a small percentage behind?

So what's happening with the rest of his energy? He's up there twiddling his thumbs?
(Laughs) Not easy to do, twiddling thumbs in the afterlife. Actually, there's tons of work - certainly classrooms and doing exercises, you're helping other people - you might have a variety of life tasks that you get glimpses of in your dreams, escorting dead people from Earth back to their natural state, whatever your work might be - it always has to do with energy transfer.

When Richard's asleep, is the greater part of him doing other work?
It's work that requires being able to fire on all engines. (The work of locating souls) it's essentially someone comes over and describes an energy pattern to you, because everyone has their own energy pattern, it's like describing a color. "It's

got a little orange in there, a little green and purple and a spot here," and you as the examiner, identify the color pattern, then shoot out into the universe, like a thread that connects to that color pattern and you pull it in. It all happens in a split second, but basically "Oh, you're looking for Larry" and *zoom* you're pulling Larry in. And Larry is, let's say, their deceased husband, who, for whatever reason, has been missing.

Mm-hmm.
That's just one of things Richard's doing; there's other work in other realms.

Tell us about that.
There are other planes of existence. There are a couple of religions who talk about it - Hindu is one – which examine a myriad of planes. There are various locations throughout the Universe where you can wind up, your spirit can zoom out into the deeper reaches of space, then zip through a worm hole and you wind up in another universe, next to our universe. And that universe has different rules - not that rules of science are different rules, but other rules; the energy pattern is different.

People communicate differently, etc. These other planes of existence have a myriad of possibilities. It's like (those who describe a visit) in the Life Library where you're able to see multiple streams of energy and it looks to you like you're picking up a book. You open the book up and see different patterns of a person's life, different chapters. They come to you as visuals, but basically they're just comprised of energy streams. We normally have three dimensions, there we might have 27 dimensions. The 14th dimension might have a whole universe of people, and the 24th might have another universe of people - of groups, comprised of a particular energy pattern.

So this soul living as Richard, what's he involved in? Is he in many different dimensions?
It depends what he's doing that particular day. Because when you're outside of Earth time, you're outside of time - if you think of time as a curve or a ball, and you're outside of it and you want to stick your finger in on the far side, you can also stick a finger in the near side, and if you think of the circle as the time line you can be in the fourth century and in the 20th century simultaneously.

So is there something he's involved in that's taking his energy right now?
When a conflict shows up between two individuals he tries to help resolve it – let's call him an Energy Diplomat. When he's needed somewhere he's called and helps out with that energy, then he's called to another realm and helps out with that energy… Diplomat of Energy is a good way to call it.

So are you involved with sending him out? Aware of what he's doing?
I'm aware of everything he does, because he's my primary responsibility - but it's not like I'm sending him on missions. If he comes to me and wants advice, it's

easy to share in his journey, but it's more observational. You could ask "What am I doing while Richard's off having these adventures of a lifetime?" Truth is, you're always connected and you're always experiencing somebody else's energy when you take responsibility for them, you're experiencing it at the same time.

Is he aware of what you're doing as well?
No. It's a one way filter. When he gets to a certain point, he can experience this, he's not there yet.

THE PAST LIVES OF MY SPIRIT GUIDE

He wants to know more about you. How long have you been with him?
Those 6-8 pre-Earth lives, since the time his energy was brought together in a very clever way. It was brought together millennia ago.

Did you exist before he did?
Yes, I was there when he was created. The experience is almost like when you get to the end of school, you have your graduation ceremony, but instead of four years, it may have been four hundred thousand years, and everyone's throwing confetti, and you're given your diploma - which is a new born soul.

"Your diploma is Richard," knowing this is what you've been working for - and knowing you're going to take care of this little baby soul for the next four hundred thousand years or whatever... Listen, it doesn't feel long like that all, because it's outside of time.

Where was Richard's soul energy before his 'inception?'
It's an unusual process of energy combination, and if you want to think about it from a human point of view, you have a mother and father, let's call *it mother and father* energy. Way off in the upper realms they take some clay, and the two of them work on the clay, it's a tiny little piece of clay. They add in bits of energy, almost like a mosaic of energy, and within that teeny weeny little piece there might be pieces of information they've added or put in there.

They take pieces of themselves, each sharing, and they put it in that little energy packet of a new soul and *whoosh* off it goes. Then it's cared for by other energy systems, which you might think of as midwives, in a hospital-like environment. Nurses taking care of babies, and eventually as the energy progresses and accumulates things, and depending how it's put together, it sort of bounces around and picks up more things, and picks up more information like an egg growing exponentially. You've created the DNA and now the DNA is telling it what to do, and eventually it gets to the point where it's this child spirit.

NOTE: In Newton's books his clients refer to "midwives" as entities who look after new souls after they're created.

And at that point your spirit guide shows up; "I've just graduated from my millennial journey, here we go. We're going to work on this together," and then off you go. Some spirit guides have more than one soul to look after, they have two or three, even more. The people they're guiding don't know that, because that could be a source of angst. By and large the system is one spirit guide and one soul. There are all kinds of variations, in this case, I was assigned this peanut and I've been keeping an eye on him for a long time.

How long?
Millennia.

Have you ever incarnated on Earth?
Yes; with him. I was there to help him - just to be there to be a guide, because it was a request.

You mean like you went through the whole birth process?
I was his father. It was a question of him asking me "Can't you help me on this one?" And I did. (In my previous session I stated he'd been my grandfather.)

So when your student graduates, what do you do then?
You can continue on and take another one; that's what I'll do - I'll take on another soul. As to my own spirit guide, he's now a non-reincarnating individual who is serving on somebody's Council of Elders. Those individuals are no longer caught up in the day-to-day of helping a person along. If you look at members of the spirit council, ones on the panel are non-reincarnating, underneath are spirit guides, because even though they're not reincarnating, they're in the mix of it on a daily basis – and under that are spirits, or humans.

THE SOURCE, THE ULTIMATE BLISS ENERGY CALLED GOD

And above the council?
Then you're getting closer to the Divine source of all things - I want to say there are two or three steps between. When people are before the council they feel closer to God, or some kind of divine source, but it's a little bit more complicated, there are more levels. A few more steps.

The final step is related to ultimate bliss kind of energy of purest form. Let's just call it that. And radiating out from that, is all this other stuff. It's almost like cells trying to find their way back to the source, if you want to look at it like a science fiction episode. Souls trying to get back to the source. Think of it as the Big Bang, when the Universe expands, all those things travel at this rate out to the end of the Universe, and some point they're going to all suck themselves back in again, that's just the nature of the Universe; the same is true about the energy source that creates souls. They wind up dispersing in the Universe and then they want to get back - and they do it through experience.

MY SOUL GROUP

Let's talk about Richard's soul group.
Richard's group is teachers, responsible for classes, and you can't really access them all at the same time because they're working. It's like most soul groups; you can visit them in their classroom, and you can find them in garden or lounge setting, so you can experience them there with downtime. But teachers, the level he's gotten to, the teachers are busy; I can't put it any other way. They have a tendency to be alone and just focus on their work.

Any impending connections?
Depends on factors. This work he's doing now on the afterlife is going to connect them up, because they're going to be like-minded and recognize his pattern - which is how you recognize people.

Richard's not supposed to know about certain things because it's like a puzzle. Richard's getting as much of the puzzle as he's supposed to get; he has to figure out the rest, because of course, that's the magic and wonderment and the clever complication of life. Which is what these amazing, unusual connections that people call *coincidence* are; actually they're elaborately and cleverly designed. The amount of work that goes into that design is monumental - but you don't want to point someone on the exact path they're supposed go on, because the cleverness is they'll discover it later.

Understood.
The thing he's been talking about; all action and thought and art are energy, and the idea of putting professors and scientists under hypnosis to pass knowledge to the planet is a good idea. It's a wonderful idea - the classrooms he's visited where people were cleaning energy systems; it's a fascinating topic. It's the idea that we have energy systems that travel with us through lifetimes, and those energy systems retain all the memories of our past lives, so Richard's past lives are carried with him in these sort of geometric energy packets that travel with you through life, they're like the ball bearings of life which can be accessed in times of need.

They contain millennia of experience and help you through life. But the energy packets[124] pick up negative energy as you go through life, so when you go back (to life between lives) you clean them up and have them taken into the shop to be serviced, so to speak. Those kinds of revelations and interesting insights are worth further examination.

---

[124] Sophia Kramer mentioned these energy packets in her session, noted previously.

THE LIFE PLANNING SESSION

Let's go to Richard's original life planning session.
(Seeing myself in front of a group of people) He's talking about what his life's going to be, and how he's going to do this 'outside the box' idea of helping people energy-wise through filmmaking - that's his gambit, and then he's working on the details. (My wife) Sherry's there, she's very playful with him, and it's agreed she's going to be the grounding factor in his life and they'll have children together. The affiliates are all there; his dad, brothers, they're all talking about what they're going to be doing, dad's the architect, he's a little bit of the architect at this as well.

Your dad's involved with the planning?
(Switches to Richard's point of view) Yes, because his eternal spirit's always there and we've always been affiliated. He's the architect, the guy who puts energy into physical things, takes energy and makes it into something physical. He's pointing out to me being a writer is also like being an architect, an architect of story using words. We're discussing the highlights; how I'll try to take energy and help people through filmmaking, music, everything else; painting, writing.

How did you decide it was time to incarnate?
A discussion with Rayma - "What's the next thing going to be?" which led to this session; you go through examinations with your loved ones, your soul group. You talk about the myriad of things you could do and be doing. The idea (of the planning session) is to get together with affiliated soul groups, and everybody including Rayma adds their own two cents and says "Oh, I got the perfect person for you."

They pull them in and "This is how we'll do this connection, I'll play this role," and you help them as well, saying "Tell you what, I'll play this role for you guys and I'll help you figure out this angle," and these million particles of energy are set in motion and hopefully, it all plays out - and incredibly it does.

Is there an advisor or being higher than Rayma?
In my case we're working it out ourselves, we're all capable of doing so, it's not like we're asking permission. Sometimes people ask "Would it be alright if I did this?" In our case we see ourselves as experienced souls and trust each other; when we say we're going to pull it off, we will pull it off.

Any other choices of lives?
It was my affection for my dad - for Charlie - that I'd figure out a way to show up. And my mom. I knew we'd have another wonderful adventure together, I feel it was just the most natural decision. We didn't go to the library and search for different lives - it's like I'm beyond that step, I can tie all the dots together and then go to Rayma and run it by him. His attitude towards me is "You already know how to do this stuff, you can figure it out, what's best for you, what do you think?"

A VISIT TO THE COUNCIL OF ELDERS

Rich wants to know about his council. Can you describe the scene?
I'm in Rayma's consciousness looking at Richard standing in front of his council, like the last time we were here (the previous session when Richard addressed the council), and I'm seeing it from Rayma's point of view. Richard is standing in front, kind of eager and shy and at the same time, clever and funny, but maybe a little too much in his head thinking he's clever and funny.

NOTE: In this moment, I had the very odd sensation of seeing myself from another person's point of view. In the previous visit to the council from the chapter "Vanum Populatum," I felt as if there was a buzz in the room, anticipating my presence there. At some point, I said something funny, and I thought everyone in the room roared with laughter. But now in this session, seeing that same moment from my spirit guide's point of view was humbling – I saw myself from his vantage point in the room, and when it got to the point where I thought everyone roared with laughter, it was actually a smattering of chuckles. I had the thought, "He's excited to be here, but we've been coming here for a long time."

But still... The council finds him amusing. But they've known him for a long time, we've been up here to do this quite a few times, and it's always entertaining. Certainly they appreciate him, because you don't get a lot of entertainment up here and the idea of having someone with his sense of humor and his point of view is refreshing let's say…

How many members?
I want to say 11; initially I saw 8, but I want to say there are 3 alternates hovering behind.

Does the council number change?
Yes. With age.

Let's go to a council visit before the American Indian. The Doctor in Boston.
How many people do I see this time? Seven. He picked up one more since then. The admonition about this life as a Doctor is, "Gee, that lifetime wasn't as much fun as you normally have," because he was serious, his persona wasn't like he normally is. Even as the Native American he was lighter, more fun. But in this Doctor life, the weight of his work wore heavily on him.

It's kind of "Well, so what did you learn from that (life) other than how not to tell a joke?" In that council session, it's about him sharing the energy of helping people, or curing people, and how that affected him and to see how that was important and connect to it. Also to have a family; it was one of the few times he's had a full family - and just the wonderfulness of that, being able to experience other humans being raised and experiencing life. So that was a wonderful journey and how much he appreciated that. I'm trying to look at this 8th council member in his most recent session.

Let's ask Rayma.
Rayma's saying it's a healing person on the council; somebody connected to Luana and her healing class. I'm also getting the 8 people are in front now, the three people behind are people he knows, but they're hidden so he can't see them - Luana might be in there, back row of the council.

Who's there?
(Identifying the various members of my Council of Elders as I saw them) From left to right; Healer, Teacher, Orator, Energy of Art; as in Artistry, Painting, Theater and all that. What is that? Four? Then comes Courage, five. Humor or the energy of humor, of comedy.

All male?
We have a mixture. Humor is male, a kindly face, I've known him forever. The last one is Music. Then an energy transfer specialist. Someone who specializes in the transference of energy from one entity to another. These are all abilities Richard has access to. By the way, comedy and tragedy are the same thing. I'm hearing this again, it's faster between your ears and your lips with comedy, but tragedy has the same affect in terms of energy. Making people laugh is a quicker way to heal them, but people experience tragedy through your art is another way to heal them, it just takes longer - not any better, not any worse.

Not any deeper?
No, when you're talking about energy repair in somebody that's damaged and you have the ability to make them laugh, you have an instant repair. It's like a flat tire that gets inflated instantly. When you repair somebody by showing them the damage, they cry and go through a catharsis, it takes a little bit longer, but the repair is the same. It's just laughter is a faster way at healing people. As they say, "Dying is easy, comedy is hard."

A DEFINITION OF SACRED ENERGY

I'll ask for a piece of advice in his life today.
To consider what Sacred Energy means, what energy might be sacred. If you can phrase it in that way, you don't have to lose your sense of humor, but you can examine things from a different point of view. Try to allow for the Sacred more in your life. Not in terms of the church, but in terms of your honoring and paying homage to the energy within.

Can you give an example?

It has to do with when you're about to create something. When you go to say a prayer, you put yourself in a position of prayer. You might go to a church and kneel down and go through all the accoutrements to get to the prayer and the effectiveness of the prayer is stronger because you've focused your energy into that moment. You can say a prayer anywhere, driving a car, people pray all the time - when they're on a roller coaster, "Ah! Don't kill me!" When you allow yourself to have the focus to make it Sacred, it allows you to become more connected to the prayer. If your working environment is cacophony and you're figuring "I'll fix this later," you haven't put yourself in the Sacred, in that church like atmosphere; Equipoise.[125] The tip; bring the Sacred into your life on a daily basis, and within your relationships. There's something very miraculous about being with whoever you are with on the planet. Find the sacred in that, instead of the profane.

Let's give Richard a last chance to see if he has any questions of you, Rayma.

(From Richard's point of view) This has been such a vast revelation of knowledge I feel like a child walking into a candy store with a million pieces of candy, "What am I supposed to do with all this?" "Oh, it's your job to pass this along to the rest of the planet." I'd like to pay homage to everybody assisting and to Scott for taking us on this journey. As well as to pay homage to Rayma and others who generously showed up to help make sense of what I'm saying.

I'm speaking out loud and my brain repeatedly tries to question it, so thanks to Richard for allowing me to speak spontaneously. It's not easy, because his mind is always editing. Just say with great awe and inspiration and praise, thank everyone for sharing this special wisdom and knowledge and let's hope I'm capable of fashioning it in such a way to benefit others. That is why we're here - to help others on the planet, to find their true selves and overcome obstacles, emotional and energetically.

I'd like to ask Rayma to show Rich a final message today.

Just showing Richard what Sacred Art means and giving him a visual so when he's in a space where he tries to create, he'll connect to that. If you follow the Sacred in your art, it'll come out and whether it wins awards or not isn't important, what is important is the energy.

As you said "if you make something beautiful, it doesn't matter whether anyone sees it or not."

It's the energy of creation; you turn it into existence and it reverberates throughout the Universe.

---

[125] State of being balanced or in equilibrium, usually connoting something that is a product of counterbalancing. Wikipedia.

So that's what he needs to focus on. Creating the sacred.
Creating Sacred art. Please remind him.

During this second session, I felt I could access everything I'd seen or heard previously, everything from my past session, as well as all my memories, thoughts, opinions. It felt incredibly authentic, and I was surprised by information downloaded by it. I can say unequivocally, I don't talk the way Rayma talks. In my conscious state, I'm convoluted, unclear and all over the map. Perhaps I should spend more time in a hypnotic state!

But my second session had a much more profound impact on me. For starters, I'd been able to go back and find Luana once again. She was sitting in her healing class, just as before. She even mocked me; "What, are we on a *talk show*?" (Her sense of humor, honestly, not mine.) During this journey I was able to find Luana twice. Her old pal B.J. once asked me "Why you? I knew her for 50 years. Why wouldn't she return to see her close friends?" Well, the good news is, she's waiting for her pals who *will* see her again and keeping an eye on them as well. From where I stood, it looked to me like she was having a hell of a time. Pardon me, having a heaven of a time.

The other profound message I got was to consider the Sacred in all things, including art, including energy, even this book. I can only hope it reaches the people it's supposed to reach, and affect those that need its message. So in a sense, my documentary began as a journey into the research as presented by various people about reincarnation and how it's physically done, and wound up with an in depth interview with my spirit guide Rayma, who's lived many more lifetimes than I have, and has some interesting things to say about the future of the planet, and how we can ensure we get there together. I didn't plan for myself to be the final interview for this book, it just worked out that way. A year had passed between my first session and beginning this book, it felt necessary to go back and revisit what I thought I'd learned. And the second time around, I got a chance to see multiple lives and multiple choices about why I came back. We all go through these choices. The trick is to stop and examine during this life why we've made them.

While in Tibet, I attended a festival near Mt. Kailash celebrating the Buddha. I took a prayer flag, wrote names of friends and loved ones on it, included a photograph, and turned it over to a monk who put it in with the thousands of other prayer flags donated to make up the large Christmas tree of flags they put up during the ceremony. The mountain of flags had to be 40 feet high. Some hours later, I offered to help put up some of the flags onto the pole, and as I stood there pulling out flags, the one I had written on appeared in my hand. Out of all the flag strands, all the people putting up flags, I'd found the very one I'd created and took this picture of it.

It reminds me that there are no coincidences.

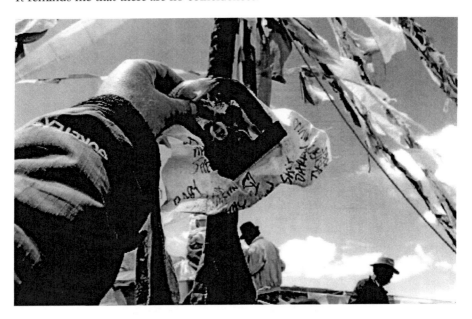

The good news is we're all going back home one day, we're all going to find our loved ones and understand why we were on this journey together. So for now, why not just sit back and enjoy the ride?

EPILOGUE
WHAT'S IT ALL ADD UP TO?

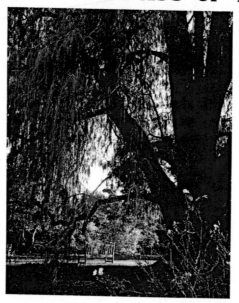

Warren Buffet, one of the richest people on the planet, was interviewed recently about the secret to his success. "Unconditional Love," he said, "the most powerful force on the planet." His father had given him unconditional love – it was a love that allowed him to fail, to get up and try again.[126]

How does all of this affect how we approach our own lives? If we know energy lives forever, that our souls live forever, that we're on the journey we chose to be on, how does that help us "make it through the night?" In an effort to connect some dots, please allow me to recap:

[126] Huffington Post 7-8-10 "The Best Life Advice I've Ever Received."

1. *Souls don't die.*

We've been around for millennia, our souls continue on for millennia. In between lives we are fully conscious, with all of our memories intact. Yes, our bodies die, our loved ones depart from us in this life. But we reconnect with them in the Afterlife.

2. *After death we return to our soul group, where we recognize those we've been reincarnating with for eons.*

There's anywhere from 3-25 people in our individual group and we usually plan our next life with these same folks. We share laughs and memories of the life just lived and eventually plot with them our next adventure. We may even recognize them during this lifetime; usually identified with the thought "I felt like I always knew this person the moment I met them," or "I knew we would marry."

3. *In between lives, we all have a life planning session where we choose our next life; we are able to pick and choose what kind of life we want to lead for various reasons, as well as choose our parents.*

"Why would I choose those people who've made my life miserable?" is a familiar refrain. The answer is that you chose them so that you could be where you are today. Either far, far away from them - which is a gift in some cases, or their influence had directly put you in the place you're supposed to be on the planet. It puts a different spin on your parents behavior when you consider you chose them because of it. As well as why your own children chose you.

4. *We each have our own "council of elders" who oversee our lifetimes, and engage with us in Socratic debate about how we did.*

Everyone has a council of elders, and everyone goes to see them at least twice; once upon our return so they can help assimilate all the lessons from that lifetime, and once again just before we take another trip into human form. They don't sit in judgment; rather they help you discern your path. Usually there are 6-12 people on any given council; it seems the younger souls have fewer.

5. *No humans are born without a soul, and we don't arrive at our chosen body until the fourth month (or sometimes later).*

Consciousness is something we've retained from our life between lives. Some kind of veil, or filter, prevents us from remembering those previous lives. However, through the process of deep hypnosis, we're able to bypass these filters and access these previous memories. The idea that we don't join the body until the fourth month would be controversial to advocates who believe life begins at conception. The human animal life may begin at conception, but the spiritual life does not.

6. *We don't reincarnate as other animals.*

Each species comes back with in its own pantheon; i.e. birds of a feather, fish in the sea, and animals on land can swap places with those in their group, but not within other groups. To the concept of being reborn in a "lower life form" as a result of negative karma - that's not what is reported. All life forms are sacred; there are no pejoratives when it comes to life. However, its reported you can access your animal friends at any time in the life between lives – they're an energy pattern as well, and can spend hours playing fetch once again.

7. *When we return to our home base, with our soul group, all actions and effects are left behind - we return to a pure state where we enjoy a world without pain, sin or suffering. There is no hell per se, nor a Satanic like region or persona.*

Those who've caused pain, sin or suffering experience the pain they inflicted fully – as if they were the person being hurt during their life review. Afterwards they may choose (or it's decided for them) to be isolated from others in order to learn from their mistakes. There is no Satan or hell per se. Once you depart this plane, you no longer have access to the negativity here, or those who might perpetrate it. (For those Satanists out there, sorry, don't mean to offend.) According to the thousands who've journeyed into the afterlife, there's no evil waiting for us. But we may experience our own form of hell based on how we've treated other human beings.

8. *The process of reincarnation is planned by us, not subject to karma, past mistakes, or past injustices. People choose to be gay, choose to be crippled, or choose to be blissful depending on their spiritual depth.*

We don't travel up or down in any fashion, going from peasant to rich person, or unhappy soul to happy soul. Free will is the law of the Universe, and it's up to us who we want to return as, or even if we want to reincarnate. But inevitably, the pull of helping your loved ones and friends, brings us back time after time. Our life choices are up to us. That includes sexuality, physical type, body shape, etc. We may choose to struggle with these issues in order to progress spiritually, or to help those around us to progress. Those who live on the fringes of society are frequently older souls who chose to be there.

9. *Bad experiences, including suicide, murder, mayhem and other events are frequently worked out in advance, with the agreement of all souls involved.*

They claim there's no such thing as random violence. This may sound controversial, but according to the research, pretty universal. When examining a life between life session, we get an opportunity to see those details, however heinous or upsetting, to be true.

10. *Our friends in our soul group frequently show up as pals in this life, relatives, brothers, sisters, loved ones or even as adversaries.*

As mentioned, Judas claimed Jesus came to him and asked him to turn him over to the Romans as a favor. "If you truly love me, you'll do this for me." There are many reasons to be on the planet, we benefit from all our own experiences, but the main role might be one of servitude.

11. *Our progression in the afterlife can be charted, in part, based on what color we see ourselves as - the earlier souls are closer to white, and through the spectrum, they wind up into the violet realm. But there is no hierarchy.*

As Jimmy Quast put it; "No one gets to hoard the jelly beans." The idea of someone being smarter, better, richer, happier, more famous, more revered, more anything is just not the case. You are the perfect self you're meant to be. All paths are sacred, and none is judged lesser than another. Just older.

12. *We all have a soul, spirit guide or "Guardian Angel," sometimes more than one.*

Every one of us has a spirit guide who has agreed to watch over all of our incarnations. It gives new meaning to the sacrifice one does at the service of others - can you imagine becoming a mentor to a soul for all of their lifetimes? But the journey many of us are on is to eventually be a guardian angel (spirit guide) for another soul; no time like the present to start treating others like they might be a future candidate.

13. *All of this movement and planning is based on energy.*

Every thought, action, word or deed contains it, every emotion as well. Treat it with sacred intent, whether praying for deliverance, or to help another soul. If you think it, believe it, pray for it, sing it, act it or create it, you've put that personal energy out into the Universe. It can help, heal, or in negative cases, harm others.

14. *There are other Universes and places we can reincarnate. Some religions have spoken of them, various planes in different dimensions Religion is a construct that mirrors the afterlife.*

Earth is the best school, the best playground, the best place to advance our souls. "You'll learn more in one day of tragedy on Earth, then perhaps 5,000 years on another, simpler planet," according to one interview. The argument has been raised, "There aren't enough souls to reincarnate. Where'd the new souls come from?" According to Newton's patients, there are other places to reincarnate and new souls are reportedly being born. When we graduate from our many lifetimes, the graduation ceremony includes being rewarded with (and offering to guide through many lifetimes) a new soul.

15. *Love and compassion turn out to be not just religious concepts, but words that explain how the Universe actually works; from energy transfer to why we choose a particular life.*

Love is the wheelwork of nature, and that attraction and energy is what keeps us going. Compassion is part of the fabric as it's included in many examples of what we give our loved ones by reincarnating by their side. The Golden Rule is actually golden for a reason, because it represents how the Universe works. Loving your neighbor as yourself, nature as yourself, your fellow beings on all levels as yourself, turns out to be not only a spiritual maxim, but a physical one as well.

16. *Religion is a man-made experience based on our god like nature.*

In light of this research, world religions seem to be echoing the same thing; in the afterlife we have eternal qualities, and experience a heaven-like state of bliss. And while we're on Earth, we try to recreate or relive that experience. One could say we're "trying to get back to the Godhead," or "return to God." They're the same. Was Jesus the son of God? Aren't we all? Was Moses or Mohammed the chosen prophet? Aren't we all?

Oddly enough, the angel Gabriel was the one who brought the word of God to the Prophet Mohammed in a cave. He's also the angel who brought news to Mary, and predicted the birth of John the Baptist. Could they all be the same Angel Gabriel? If he exists outside of time, why not? The founder of Mormonism, Joseph Smith, had a visitation from men "dressed in white" who dictated a vision of the afterlife to him, L. Ron Hubbard believed he'd seen another planet from which we return to Earth via Scientology. It seems they're all talking about the same thing when they refer to the Kingdom of Heaven or even to Buddha's journey on the night of his enlightenment to see "non-reincarnating deities."

Religion expresses the inexpressible, examines the unexamined, and finds truth in the nature of all things. Science aspires to take the same journey, by making logical sense of what we are doing on the planet, how we got here, and where we are going. For those who believe that life ends in death, that's not what's reported. For those who think the stress of this lifetime is based on karma from a previous one; that too doesn't bear up under this form of scrutiny. Forgiveness, compassion and love for all people and things appears to be the universal law of the Universe.

17. *We have both an animal ego and a spiritual ego.*

According to this research, we started incarnating on Earth millennia ago. Perhaps when humans became upright or adept; our spiritual energy melded with the human's, and thus began consciousness. Perhaps this event coincided with the formation of societies 60,000 years ago and is our "missing link."

Human life appears to be an agreement between the animal and spiritual ego. That fact helps to underline why people act a certain way, and could have a profound influence on the criminal justice system – if a person is struggling in this life with animalistic tendencies is there a way of examining a healing process that's not "Clockwork Orange[127]" but based on helping souls discover their purpose? As mentioned, in Holland, they've already [128]begun to bring in psychics and past life regressionists to help cure career criminals.

18. *Curing and healing people is part of the work done by others in the Afterlife.*

People choose their lifetimes before coming here to continue their work in a particular field. Musicians may return to further their music knowledge, perhaps explaining child prodigies like Mozart and others. Doctors and Nurses are involved with healing energy transfer, and may have had many lifetimes where they continued their practice. Just the way Tibetan lamas might spend a lifetime studying esoteric practices, and then remember them in their ensuing lifetime, we can all tap into the knowledge of our previous lifetimes to help with our current one.

19. *There are no coincidences.*

What appears to be a matter of amazing coincidence, upon examination, turns out to be an incredible planned sequence, like a complex 3D chess or "Second Life" game being played on multiple planes where each move affects the other players. As a butterfly's wings in a rain forest may cause a hurricane in Asia, everything can be linked in cause and effect if one looks long and hard enough. And by the way, is the reason you've picked up this book.

20. *You are doing pretty much what you set out to do.*

Time and again, people report the spiritual journey they're on was laid out in advance. This is annoying for anyone with a remote control - we all have the inclination to change the channel, to want to change our circumstance, get richer quicker - but the answer is: "You're doing fine, you're on the right path, relax." As hard as your path may seem, you're on it for a spiritual reason.

21. *This research is the tip of the iceberg.*

For those who are interested in finding their soul's purpose – the reason they chose to be here on the planet – I can't think of a more effective way. Here's some collected insights from the therapists I interviewed:

People come in because there may be a relative who recently died, or emotional trauma from losing a child. This work is not to supplant therapy they should receive from a licensed trained professional; it's intended to provide them with answers about their inner being. One of the things clients don't understand until they experience it is that

---

[127] The book by Anthony Burgess mocks criminal rehab in the future where prisoners are reprogrammed.

[128] The Telegraph 22 Nov. 2010 "Dutch prisons use psychics to help prisoners contact the dead."

there is a dual nature to all of us. We have our brain ego if you will, and we have a soul ego, and when they are combined it creates one personality and one lifetime.

- Michael Newton

Someone can have a strong religious belief that doesn't include reincarnation, but when you take someone through one of these sessions, they have this mind boggling experience - it's a visceral experience on a soul and body level – they emerge knowing this to be true. It's far beyond a concept or belief. That's profound. One other common occurrence is a feeling of reconnecting to the whole. To know you and I are of the same essence makes it much more difficult for me to cause you harm, because it's harming me and the whole as well. That's a message for the entire planet; how we cause harm to others. It's more difficult to do knowing we are all the same. I'd love to see everyone have the opportunity to go through one of these sessions. It's wonderful that it's not a dogma, it's not a religion, but it's open to everyone.

- Paul Aurand

I believe we are spiritual beings that live on this Earth. We're not Earthly beings who happen to be spiritual, but the other way around. So for me, this past life work, soulful work, is about that fact that at our core, we're this beautiful diamond and the mud that covers it are experiences in other lifetimes we've encountered. And we create these negative beliefs we have about ourselves, whether it's shame or self-hatred or unworthiness, and sometimes we have to go all the way back to the beginning - our past lives - to wash away the mud so we can uncover the beautiful diamond we are. Until you get to the source of it, you're going to be in conflict with nature until you find the source of the diamond within you.

- Debbie Haynie

Always wisdom is uppermost in mind. We choose to incarnate to harvest wisdom from the lifetime, to gain direct experience and knowledge so that we are improved as beings, so that we are expanded as beings, so that we have more wisdom, understanding and compassion.

- Colleen Page-Joy

There's this very bright light everywhere I look; I'm part of it. He's showing me I'm part of a universal plan, I'm part of that light and it's everywhere, there's nowhere in the universe there isn't this light. He says "That's what you're working with, keep it as part of you and bring it back." We need to know there's nothing else but light and love. The work we're doing (as hypnotherapists) is about light, because it opens us up to understanding. We're on a mission to clarify and create more light and love and it's available to everyone; all we have to do is open ourselves to it. The light is clear and cleansing, loving and peaceful. Eventually when we become light all the other things go; sadness and such. It's very healing.

- Morrin Bass

To date it's the single most important modality I can offer anyone. It gives them a sense of their immortality, of the importance of their life and journey, and it gives a sense of belonging to something greater than themselves. It's not a gifted psychic telling you who you are or what you've been, or going to a "Channeler" to tell you your past and background; it's experiential, the clients become their own channel. After every single client has an LBL, they aren't the same – some part of them has changed in a positive way and it's a resource that remains for them long after their Life between Lives journey is complete.

- Chanda Nancy Berlatsky

I think traditional belief systems are breaking down all over the world; people are looking for something more, for a greater understanding of themselves, rather than being told by other people what to believe. If you can look at what you have within, that's got to be the real stuff because it's your own. If you can tap into that, have access to that, it's very empowering. The world is picking up pace and if we can have something that's centering, like an awakening and understanding of your immortal identity, that seems to be the most centering you could ever have. The more people discover the beautiful compassion and wisdom we hold within, that's got to be good for the planet.

- Peter Smith

A CALL TO ARMS (EMBRACING ONES)

Imagine if one day scientists, doctors, philosophers could all do life between life classrooms? People who understand physics could learn from the classes on energy transfer, doctors could sit in on classes about the healing light of the Universe; philosophers could examine and ask questions about this other, primary world that would benefit our current one. Religious leaders could clarify what their purpose on the planet is, and why they chose a life to help people spiritually (if they haven't already). It could cause advancements in human science, psychology, medicine, conservation as well as in renewable energy and its resources, as well as helping humanity to fulfill its purpose.

Those who take a journey into this other world, come away from it profoundly changed. They start to see the many connections their lives have to offer - whether how a childhood friend first put you on your pathway, or how a sense of knowing someone from the past can be achieved by merely shaking someone's hand. As Paul Aurand put it "hard for me to want to harm you when I see how we're all spiritually connected."

People under hypnosis say they discover the Universe is run on "love;" failing another word in the English language, it's the best they can find to describe it. Love is the ether that bonds the universe, the gravity or hidden dark matter that binds all elements together. A sea of atoms of energy particles we navigate every day, but its pulse, its heart, is love – towards our fellow humans, towards nature, towards the planet, towards the universe. It's been echoed in all the great tales of literature, of myth and legend, throughout our time together on the planet. We've become used to our belief science can solve the problems of humanity, when actually the true force that can solve the problems of the planet is our willingness to participate in the love we all innately have for it and each other.

And this applies to every curmudgeon you've ever met, every cranky, unhappy, miserly person – once they're off the planet, they return to their blissful selves, where they get the opportunity to see how connected we all are, and how they've missed the golden opportunity to revel and enjoy life from a compassionate point of view.

Someone asked Michael Newton why he thought this information was becoming evident now - the question begs to be asked; for all the years we've had civilization on the planet, why reveal it now?

He doesn't know the answer. Perhaps this information has always been accessible; we didn't have the ability to decipher it. Perhaps it's the abuse of drugs and pharmacological "cures" that change the course of one's soul path, perhaps people in the afterlife are trying to warn us.

I think it may be to convince people that reincarnation does exist, and therefore, we must protect the planet for our return. The interview with the gentleman who said he was a "hybrid" – someone who incarnates on another planet as well as Earth – claimed he and his fellow hybrids have come here to enhance people's consciousness. (I jokingly asked him when I met him for lunch, if it wasn't "To Serve Man," a reference to the infamous Twilight Zone episode where the textbook aliens left behind turned out to be a cookbook. He laughed.) But according to his interview, over the next seven years, consciousness will change on Earth. Whether true or not, the future depends on a multitude of factors; of chess games and our spirit guides controlling the board.

The internet has connected us in ways we never thought possible - which mirrors the afterlife in the connections we already have, spiritually, energetically, between ourselves. The phenomenon of social networks is that they mirror the life between lives; we're all connected, can reach anyone anywhere at any time.

The ability to retain information in a computer mirrors our ability to retain information. The transference of energy through ones and zeroes mirrors the transference of energy that occurs on a daily, or moment to moment basis. Is it possible that consciousness, or the spirit world is the same? That we carry engrams of energy around with us, like hard drives floating in the ether of space, so we can refer to past lives and experiences?

I got a text the other day from a friend who was sitting in "Les Deux Magots" café in Paris, when he chatted up the leggy singer sitting at the next table. The conversation drifted around to past life regression, and she said "You should talk to my friend Rich Martini." Turns out my two friends, both New Yorkers, had found themselves next to each other discussing the very topic of this book. I hope it engenders more meetings of the heart, and spirit.

I had a vision while working long hours on the film "Salt." I had been away from my family for a number of months, and I seriously doubted the sanity of working such long hours on someone else's creative endeavor. And then I had this vision of an orphanage in Cambodia.

Angelina Jolie supports an orphanage in Cambodia, and last year, she and her partner Brad Pitt donated seven million dollars to charity. I saw my vision as a way of making a connection between the long hours working on the film and the feeding of starving children that would result from her donations. Still, didn't make me miss my family any less. But then a few nights later, I had another vision that clarified this previous one. I saw into the future a young boy on the streets of India, a beggar, selling an illegal copy of "Salt" in a back alley. I saw how the few rupees from that sale went to feeding his family living out of box behind him. And in that visual, I saw that the creative energy of filmmaking, the wheelwork of commerce, of life itself, benefits people in ways we can't fathom.

Because it was an illegal copy, it allowed me to see the energy involved had nothing to do with creating wealth; rather, the energy was like a giant Tesla coil reaching people in ways I couldn't predict. All our endeavors spread out like an energy wave through the universe, helping people we'll never see.

Is life designed in advance? Are we all part of some elaborately plotted mini-series that runs every waking moment? Does it really matter one way or the other? We're on the planet for a reason, we have roles to play, we might as well play them as well as we can. However, that doesn't prevent me from perennially rooting for the Cubs.

When I was in high school, my art teacher told me I should be a painter, my acting teacher told me I should pursue a career in acting, and my football coach pulled me aside and told me I should coach football. When I mentioned this to Olivia she said "But you did none of those things!" and I said, "Actually, becoming a film director allowed me to do all three; paint with words and light, I usually appear in my films, and directing is coaching others into doing their best work." I can point to my own journey to say it appears I'm doing what I set out to do.

When I underwent my session, the world altered for me; if you'd like to try it, I recommend searching for the right hypnotherapist, trained by TNI if you'd like to visit previous lives and between lives. (There's a list of Michael Newton trained hypnotherapists at newtoninstitute.org).

Take a yoga class, learn how to meditate. Whatever gets you into the mindset is the right modality for you. As Pete Smith said, "Whatever book I need to find today, let it come to me" and he picked up Newton's "Journey of Souls." Trust in your higher self to guide you to the right material for you – after all, let's give him or her credit for guiding you to this one.

Once you've taken the trip it's like opening a gateway and other bits of information flow freely, information that seems to come directly from the Great Beyond; the ability to see why you chose your parents, your life situation, and to be able to further examine your soul's purpose. You see how we're all connected; energetically, spiritually – and those people putting stones in your path may be doing so at your request to experience a problem or pain, and learn from it spiritually. What better way to take the reins of life than to understand the truth of why you chose it?

My journey was complete; Luana mused she was going to another galaxy; I was able to find that galaxy, and to take a couple of mind bending trips to see her. She spoke to me in both of my sessions – each time in her unique voice. As mentioned, whether one believes they're seeing their loved one or not is beside the point, they have the profound experience of actually doing so.

And one final word from Luana. Recently, her old friend and one time paramour Dennis Hopper passed away. At her funeral, he sent the second largest bouquet of flowers I'd ever seen in my life. (The other was from Jack Nicholson, and stood opposite the one from Dennis.) When he passed away recently, I started to wonder if the two met up, but before the thought was fully formed in my head, I heard Luana say "He's here with me now." Then I saw an image of him, as a young man, about 20, and there was a golden light coming from within him, pouring out of him like light rays. I heard him say "This is amazing, man," in the way that only Dennis Hopper could say it. I then heard Luana say, clear as a bell; "He's my golden boy."

Final thought; my daughter and I were discussing God the other day – she's 7, I'm 56. We agreed upon "God is the mechanism by which we perceive the Universe – not a person, actually. We are all part of the mechanism that is God – the higher energy source for all things. That's why people say *God is love*, because God represents the unfathomable engine that creates and anchors the love between all of us."

See you on the flipside.

APPENDIX
TRAVEL TIPS ON
TOURING THE AFTERLIFE

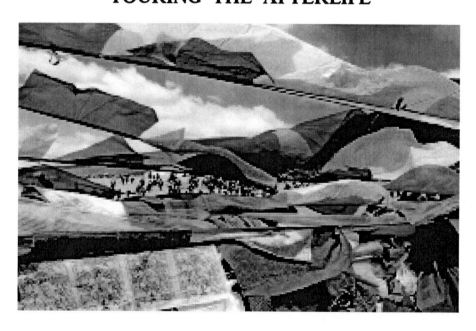

Being able to journey to the afterlife through your mind requires a certain amount of assistance, either through the help of a trained professional, or through training the mind. To help experience a trip to the Afterlife, I've included the following workbook.

PREPARING THE TRIP

Meditation

Meditation is the single most important tool to tame the mind. Here are some basic meditations.

#1. *The Breathing Meditation.* It requires the practitioner to find a place that's comfortable to sit in, a place preferably without noise (sometimes noise can be helpful), a place you won't be bothered. Just breathe deeply. Count the breaths. Breathe in and imagine that it's good energy entering and bad energy emerging. The point is, don't think, and just examine your breath for ten minutes every day.

#2. *Vase Meditation* Picture yourself under a waterfall and let the water pound your shoulders, head and back. Let the water flow down into and begin to fill your body. Let it flow to every one of your appendages. When it reaches the top, open the spigot in your toe and let the water rush out. Let out all the thoughts you've had, negative or positive. Repeat. Best performed while showering.

#3. *Walking Meditation* Buddhist monk Thich Nhat Hanh has written extensively about the effects of being present with each step you take. Memorize a path near your home. Every tree, every home you pass. Then when in another location, a crowded city perhaps, recreate in your mind the path near your home. We're on a rigorous journey into the afterlife, do a little stretching before the trip.

#4. *Tonglen* This is the meditation used by Dr. Davidson in his studies of meditation at the University of Wisconsin. Picture your ailing loved one (or the planet) in front of you. Breathe in the illness or troubles with your inward breath. As the troubles or illness comes inside of you, use the healing light of the universe to dissolve and destroy the illness. Send back into the loved one, or the planet, the newly minted healing light. Studies prove this meditation can cure depression, but it also hones the mind.

ROAD SIGNS AND SNAP SHOTS

If your purpose for taking this journey is to visit a loved one, some tools are needed.

#1. *A photograph of your loved one.* James Van Praagh recommends holding photo of a loved one before going to sleep and meditating on a question. Apparently photographs retain energy of those departed, like a slice of preserved time.

#2. *Prepare a question.* "Are you okay?" won't do. Yes, they are okay; they're home and enjoying their time there. It's like answering a cell phone in the afterlife – Formulate the question before the journey. And don't judge the response – just write whatever comes to mind down, and examine it later. Is it a message from a departed one? From your own spirit? Or a clue to bigger puzzle?

#3. *Prepare yourself for a conversation.* Prepare yourself to have a conversation with your loved one. Don't judge what you think you hear, just answer in your mind's eye and write down what you think you heard and examine it later.

CHOOSING THE RIGHT VEHICLE

#1. *Astral Projection.* The initiation is a strong buzzing sensation, and then a kind of paralysis that overcomes the body. Not to worry, that's just the sensation of lifting out of the body. If it happens, just let go. This method requires practice.

#2. *Flying around the room.* Many people report that they can see a filament of white light attached to their bodies while flying around the room, or taking a journey somewhere. Many people awake with a jolt once they've jumped back into their bodies.

#3. *Document the trip.* I'm a fan of writing it down after the experience, so whatever you saw or heard can be examined later. Sometimes you see and hear things that don't make sense for months, even years.

TAKING A TOUR OF A PAST LIFE

#1. *Get the right tour guide.* I recommend finding a hypnotist trained in the Newton Method. I've documented their work. They can help understand why you chose a past life, and why you chose this one. You can find a list of those at the Newton Institute's website.

#2. *Take the Stairs if Needed.* Many past life regressions begin with a set of stairs. Perhaps it's going backwards in time from one age to an earlier age. "Is it day or night?" "What are you wearing?" "Are you a boy or girl?" "How old are you?" You can use a hypnotherapists CD to do this kind of self-examination.

TAKING A LIFE BETWEEN LIFE JOURNEY

I don't recommend doing this alone. People can, but there may be things in your past that are disturbing or confusing. Having a well-trained therapist by your side is the wisest way to proceed.

#1. *Look for Your Spirit Guide.* Everyone has one. There may be two, as sometimes they have trainees that are learning. Your spirit guide is usually the first person to show up, to help guide you through the afterlife.

#2. *Look for your soul group.* According to Dr. Newton's research, anywhere from 3-25 people are in your primary soul group. They're people you've been reincarnating with for a long time. You'll know them when you see them.

#3. *Look for your council of elders.* It's usually from 6-12 non reincarnating individuals who are only there to help you evaluate your previous life. They also appear just prior to your return to earth, and help you examine what it is that you're setting out to do.

FLAT TIRES AND MECHANICAL PROBLEMS

People die or fall off the bus, friends change, stones fall into your path. But there are service stations along the way.

#1. *Depression.* Depression, like any problem with the body or mind, is something that needs to be addressed like any illness. What's the root cause of it? When in doubt, seek help from a professional, even if that person is your local hypnotherapist. But the roots of your depression or other mental illness may be in the spirit world. It's worth looking into to find the root cause.

#2. *Perspective* The Buddhists have an excellent way of examining reality. A car cuts you off and you want to kill the other driver. Then you see they've prevented you from running over a person you didn't see. You love the other driver. We're faced with value added attachments every day – and we usually don't have the tools to examine them with. Allow more perspective into your life.

#3. *Dents* We always have unforeseen accidents in life. One way to examine these is to remember, "I chose this life, I chose my parents, and I chose this body." Why did you make those choices? Pretend for a moment we did choose the obstacle – then what to make of it? How can it help us progress? How can we become better spiritual beings?

SOUVENIERS AND OTHER GIFTS

"He who dies with the most toys, wins." Not true. The bumper sticker should read "He who dies with the most love wins."

#1. *There's no hierarchy in the afterlife.* "No one can horde the jellybeans." I'm sorry; did you say you were famous in your past life? You made how much money? You did what with the time you spent on Earth? I'm sorry to hear that.

#2. *We're all equal.* Fame, fortune, even talent. It's irrelevant in the life between lives. Once you're back there, you won't have any mask to wear. Everything is as simple as it is in real life – without all the value added things we attach to things of vanity.

#3. *Victory Laps.* Those who seem happiest upon their return are those who've lived lives filled with compassion, those who've overcome difficult struggles on Earth. However, there's no negative judgment reserved for any life, except by those who've lived it.

CLEAN UP YOUR CAMPSITE

#1. *You're returning.* Clean up after yourself! Elect officials and support causes who guarantee plenty of fresh water and clean air and trees to create the air for your return. Renewable energy takes on a new meaning when you're coming back to use it.

#2. *Take the knowledge* that you've learned in your life and put it to use to help others. Know how to light a fire with two sticks? Teach someone else. Know how to channel energy from the Universe that can help heal people in hospices? Do that.

#3. Start thinking now; who do I want to return as? The Dalai Lama meditates four hours a day on where he's going to return. He says he already knows. Picture what kind of person you'd like to be in your next life. Ask your higher self for guidance.

RULES OF THE ROAD TO PONDER

#1. Karma is a choice, not a burden. Karma doesn't follow us like baggage. Since we have free choice in the afterlife, we decide what baggage we want to pick up in the next life.

#2. People who do bad things will be punished. There is no Satan, no hell. However, those who commit heinous acts are directed to an area where they can meditate (experience) all the negativity they've created. Worse than prison, or hell.

#3. Who dies with the most love, wins. Everyone reports a blissful state where you can reconnect with all your loved ones. No matter how bad this life gets, there will be a wonderful journey back to where we all came from. Sounds like heaven to me.

SLIDE SHOW PLEASE! LET'S RECAP

#1. Does God exist? Yes. There is a God. And no, there isn't one per se, rather an indefinable source of energy.

#2. Am I human or spirit? Both. All-in-one. One isn't better than the other; equal halves to one whole. Honor both.

#3. Do we die? Our bodies do. Our souls don't.

#4. What's the meaning of life? Trick question. The answer is; the journey you chose to go on.

HAPPY MOTORING!

"Y'all come back now, ya hear?"

RECOMMENDED READING

"Journeys Out Of the Body" by Robert Monroe

Monroe is the Godfather of "astral projection" and has written many books on the subject.

"Talking to Heaven" by James Van Praagh

I spoke to my departed pal Luana through James. The second half of this book describes schools and classes in the afterlife.

"Tibetan Book of the Dead," translated by Robert Thurman

I greatly prefer Robert Thurman's version of this document. Robert's book "Essential Tibetan Philosophy" is equally terrific.

"The Jewel Tree of Tibet," by Robert Thurman

The meditation is one that benefits your heart and soul and mind.

"Many Lives, Many Masters" by Brian Weiss

Based on patients who spontaneously regressed during hypnotherapy, Weiss was the first scientist to publish studies of PLRs.

"Yesterday's Children" by Jenny Cockell

A woman in England who kept having strong memories of an earlier life in Ireland. [129]

---

[129] Or the follow up book "Across Time and Death: A Mother's Search For Her Past Life Children" by Jenny Cockell. 1994

"Linked: How Everything Is Connected… and What It Means" By A.L. Barabasi

How clustering is one of the laws of the Universe, apparently for souls as well.

"MindScience: An East-West Dialogue" by the Dalai Lama, Robert Thurman, etc.

The Dalai Lama argues if science differs from a Buddhist doctrine, then the doctrine must be re-examined.

"Journey of Souls" by Michael Newton.

Based on over 7000 interviews with patients, he lays out a powerful case for his vision of the afterlife, and how to get there.

"Destiny of Souls" by Michael Newton

Published a few years after the first with new cases, new revelations.

"Life Between Lives" by Michael Newton

This is a workbook for the hypnotherapist who desires to learn Newton's method. A must read for serious past life regressionists.

"Memories of the Afterlife" Edited by Michael Newton

Stories submitted by hypnotherapists he's trained, includes follow ups with the patients themselves. A Must Read.

"The Holographic Universe" by Michael Talbot

The idea that holography explains much of the physical and spiritual universe as we know it.

"The Essence of Tibetan Buddhism" by Lama Yeshe

Lama Yeshe's books have clarity and a humorous approach to Tibetan philosophy; most books available to read free online through LamaYeshe.com.

"Buddhism with an Attitude" by B. Alan Wallace

UC Santa Barbara Professor and scholar B. Alan Wallace, like Robert Thurman, was a westerner who became a Tibetan monk.

"The Afterlife Experiments" Gary Schwartz with William Simon

Former scientist at Harvard and Yale explores scientific evidence of what ESP and psychic ability might be about.

"The G.O.D Experiments" by Gary Schwartz with William Simon

Science points to a "Guiding Principal" behind evolution which may be some form of consciousness.

"Good Life, Good Death" by Rinpoche Nawang Gelek

Really clear, concise examination of the Buddhist tradition of the Afterlife.

"Courageous Souls: Do We Plan Our Life Challenges Before Birth?" by Robert Schwartz

Robert contacted people through the net who felt they had chosen their difficult lives via a "life planning session" in the afterlife.

"Travels" by Michael Crichton

The author of "Jurassic Park" and "E.R.," examines the spiritual journey of his life.

"Evidence of the Afterlife" The science of NDEs by Jeffrey Long, MD with Paul Perry

A book about Near Death experiences and the results are fairly uniform.

"The Power Of Myth" by Joseph Campbell

Written with Bill Moyers, how myths cross all cultures. Some of those myths have a genesis in the life between lives.

"If I Only Knew Then… Learning From Our Mistakes" by Charles Grodin

The prolific actor, writer, pundit and humanitarian examines how mistakes might help define a person's journey through life.

My Life After Life - A Posthumous Memoir by Galen Stoller

A breath taking account written by a young boy who passed away, edited by his father who is a renowned Doctor. Amazing descriptions of between life classes.

AFTER LIFE TOUR GUIDES

Michael Newton Institute – Newtoninstitute.org
Paul Aurand – NY – Holistichealingcenter.com
Jimmy Quast – Maryland - Eastonhypnosis.com
Scott de Tamble – LA – Lightbetweenlives.com
Bryn Blankenship – North Carolina – Journeyofsouls.us
Morrin Bass – NY – NewYorkAwarness.com
Chanda Nancy Berlatsky – Sedona – Soultherapies.com
Chuck Frank – Miami - Hypnosisarts.com
Colleen Joy-Page - South Africa – Colleen-Joy.com
Peter Smith – Melbourne – LBLaustralia.com.au
Dave Parke – NYC – Coachingthesoul.com
Debra Haynie – Denver - antaskarana.com

ACKNOWLEDGMENTS

My deep appreciation to those who shared their stories with me; it's not easy to do a hypnotherapy session with a guy staring at you through a lens. To Michael Newton, and members of his Institute, especially Paul Aurand, Peter Smith and Scott De Tamble; your work is amazing. Also Chuck Frank, Jimmy Quast, thanks.

To my brothers and my concert piano playing mother Anthy, and my architect father Charlie; I couldn't have chosen better parents on the planet, and you gave me courage to follow my dreams, however unconventional they turned out to be. To Julian Baird, Dr. Fink, Robert Thurman - each one of you is a genius in your field, and though you may not have met each other, I carry your insight and wisdom, standing on "the shoulders of giants," to quote another Newton; Isaac. To Chuck Tebbets, if it's true there are no coincidences, Chuck's call proves that.

To Robert Beer, Howard Schultz, Cis Rundle, Todd Menard, Chanda Berlatsky, Patty Barrett, thank you. To Hunt Block who thought my documentary might make interesting reading. To Dr. Habib Sadeghi and his wife Sherazade; your generous support helped this come to fruition. To Gary Schwartz, who generously offered to write the Introduction. To attorney Deborah Skelley, who believed I had a book inside my footage, and my lit agent and blues harp sideman Joel Gotler and his partner Larry Becsey, synchronicity runs deep.

To Doug Martin, who designed the cool book cover, and also helped me find a rent control apt. in Santa Monica. To Nick Milo, Jeff Gross, Dick Dinges who helped me find typos, which I'm sure still exist. To Duncan Clark, Tony To, Rebecca Broussard, and Bruce Haring, all stand up pals and fierce advocates. To Francis and Ellie Coppola, Robert Towne, especially Phillip Noyce whom I feel I've known a few lifetimes. To Bob Shaye for letting me on the boat, Peter Tunney who proves you can have many lifetimes in just one.

To Elissa and Charles Grodin, amazing friend, mentor, humanitarian and Sally

Kellerman and Jonathan Krane who believed in me as a filmmaker despite evidence to the contrary. To Paul Tracey for continuing our friendship over a few lifetimes, to Dave Patlak, many pals from Northbrook, BU, the Rome Center and elsewhere – fellow compatriots all.

To Luana Anders, who continues to make things possible from the Great Beyond. Despite knowing you're still here, you're truly missed. Finally, to my wife, the amazing Sherry, my children Olivia and RJ who have joined me on this journey in this lifetime. Without your anchoring support and appreciation, I wouldn't be here in the first place, and your loving grace has kept me going throughout. And to all of you, thanks for putting up with me in this lifetime. Let's do it again... but not too soon!

PRAISE FOR "FLIPSIDE"

"Richard has written a terrific book. Insightful,
funny, provocative and deep; I highly recommend it!"

- **Robert Thurman** *("Why the Dalai Lama Matters")*

"Inspiring, well written and entertaining. The kind of book where once you have
read it, you will no longer be able to see the world in the same way again."

- **Gary E. Schwartz** *("The Sacred Promise")*

"Everyone should have a Richard Martini in their life."

- **Charles Grodin** *("If I Only Knew Then... What I Learned From Mistakes")*

ABOUT THE AUTHOR

Richard Martini graduated Magna Cum Laude from Boston University with a BA in Humanities, has a Master's degree from the USC Professional Writer's Program where he also attended the Graduate School of Cinema. He's taught film at Loyola Marymount in L.A. and the Loyola University of Chicago Rome Center. He's a free-lance author whose work has been published in numerous magazines including Variety, Premier and Inc.com. He's an award winning filmmaker who has written and/or directed both documentaries and feature films. He's made feature film comedies, dramas and a thriller. He's made documentaries in Morocco, India and Tibet featuring stories about Chicago's Mayor Daley, The Dalai Lama and Robert Thurman.

This is his first book.
For further info: BeThereNow.org or *FlipSide*thebook.com
Introduction photo by Russ Titelman, used with permission.

9 781624 670756

ABOUT THE AUTHOR

Richard Martini graduated Magna Cum Laude from Boston University with a BA in Humanities, has a Master's degree from the USC Professional Writer's Program where he also attended the Graduate School of Cinema. He's taught film at Loyola Marymount in L.A. and the Loyola University of Chicago Rome Center. He's a free-lance author whose work has been published in numerous magazines including Variety, Premier and Inc.com. He's an award winning filmmaker who has written and/or directed both documentaries and feature films. He's made feature film comedies, dramas and a thriller. He's made documentaries in Morocco, India and Tibet featuring stories about Chicago's Mayor Daley, The Dalai Lama and Robert Thurman.

This is his first book.

For further info: BeThereNow.org or *FlipSide*thebook.com

Introduction photo by Russ Titelman, used with permission.

CPSIA information can be obtained at www.ICGtesting.com
Printed in the USA
BVOW030207300513

322004BV00002B/46/P